EXCEPTIONAL

EXCEPTIONAL
THE GENTLE GIANT

ANNETTE FORRESTER

XULON PRESS

Xulon Press
555 Winderley Pl, Suite 225
Maitland, FL 32751
407.339.4217
www.xulonpress.com

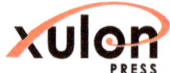

© 2024 by Annette Forrester

All rights reserved solely by the author. The author guarantees all contents are original and do not infringe upon the legal rights of any other person or work. No part of this book may be reproduced in any form without the permission of the author.

Due to the changing nature of the Internet, if there are any web addresses, links, or URLs included in this manuscript, these may have been altered and may no longer be accessible. The views and opinions shared in this book belong solely to the author and do not necessarily reflect those of the publisher. The publisher therefore disclaims responsibility for the views or opinions expressed within the work.

Unless otherwise indicated, Scripture quotations taken from the Holy Bible, New Living Translation (NLT). Copyright ©1996, 2004, 2007 by Tyndale House Foundation. Used by permission of Tyndale House Publishers, Inc.

Paperback ISBN-13: 979-8-86850-532-4
Hard Cover ISBN-13: 979-8-86850-533-1
Ebook ISBN-13: 979-8-86850-534-8

SUMMARY

This book "Exceptional the Gentle Giant," interrupts the imagination and intellect of what the world calls "Autism." It captures the essence of the transformational process of diagnosing the scientific hypothesis of the mind and perspective of Autism. This book helps to open the heart of individuals, while displaying the beauty of what our "normal" looks like. The delivery of this dialogue from Exceptional to the world unfolds in these pages as we shine light on the impossible to possible. Sharing with you, the average child and family, to the exceptional with unity, harmony, distinction, and poise for the world to see there is beauty in all of us without limitations and stigmas.

DEDICATION

This book is dedicated to the villagers! The minds that came together collectively to assist in the manifestation of what we see now. The catapulting manifestation of all your contributions; whether they were tangible, words of profound encouragement, or time well spent. Those contributions are all necessary to see a child be born, grow to adulthood, and significantly define their purpose without barriers. We love you all, and as this list is quite lengthy, we are sharing our hearts with you through these pages. Giving a huge shout out to my friends Carl Sole Jr. and Trey Paige, one love!

TABLE OF CONTENTS

Introduction xi

Chapter 1: My Pieces in Peace 1

Chapter 2: Filtering 9

Chapter 3: Finding Out 23

Chapter 4: In the Middle 39

Chapter 5: Interruption 51

Chapter 6: Expectations 67

Chapter 7: Reshaping 73

Conclusion 79

INTRODUCTION

Nothing takes the human mind by surprise anymore. There is a continual shifting of the world's view of people, places, and things. The way that it takes many deep breaths to breathe life into a dream is a testament to our human spirit. Each of us has unique things about us that allow us to embrace change by allowing faith, and not sit back passively observing.

Imagine the way we move when our nerves are rattled. For example, we are in front of a crowd of people and our heart rate may increase. These are the moments that we do some unusual things to calm us from constant daily living. Some of you may go to your room and draw beautiful pictures, or some may go in the shower and just stay in there for hours.

With others, there could be the simple act of walking to get a deeper relaxation. My friends and family, we are no different and some look on to say, "weird," well so are you. If we are doing the same to calm and cool our heads, how then do you impose judgment? We are all the same in many ways. With a plethora of diversity in backgrounds, they give us a different approach to the way life allows us to show up.

There is a path that I journey to see the outcome with huge expectations for all to gaze upon. The world has a term for this journey called "Autism." The diagnosis that interrupted my little fragile body as my years were just beginning. I can assume this has happened to many others alike. With the story of your life and mine, we are journeying together. Well, let's go! See you at the turnaround.

Exceptional

"My letter"

Here is where I somehow take this optical lens and span it from left to right. More so the left as this is how we start things and write them as well. So, with that the right is still playing itself out as my future reveals itself. As my mother and I capture these moments and translate them, everyonē will have their own way of telling their story. We are taking the hands of the adults, the friends, parents, siblings and all the villagers to our place of refuge.

I invite you to view my colorful autistic world. The one that chose me, when there was no choice for me to be here. The optics on this side are immersed in vibrant hues. We can now all look into this lens and see my incredible life. The roads we decide to travel are the ones that will carry us until we decide to get on new ones. Either way, they all have a destination, a dead end, or another road connecting for you and me to decide whether to change course or keep going. Where will this go?

With obstacles and setbacks, I am the least bit excited within these early years of this "Autism," tampering with my emotions, it's scary at times. It was moments of banging my head on the floor, that left my parents and other loved ones in a frenzy not knowing what was happening. With a fine distinction between normal and abnormal, love was pivotal in the cultivation of the soil for my growth and life within the spectrum.

The changes that happen within this writing are all so familiar to many of you and others as well I can only imagine how you will feel after reading about the revolving emotions of being an autistic individual, the typical shifts, and endless changes. It sometimes feels as if a skilled painter came in and smeared over a perfect portrait, with hopes of seeing something different.

We will try and demonstrate our world and paint the picture for you, please hold on and be mindful of the subtle nuances of social displacement. I really am a funny dude, catch me on the good days, and most of those are good because I could not care less about what others think of me. I move while creating my own beautiful displays; the ones that take your breath away.

This is where I would give most of the credit to my mom, having said that my dad is the bomb as well. He is that quiet storm type dude. I try not to cross him. My mother on the other hand, transcends such an aspiring faith that you will witness throughout these pages. I say that with so much love for her and the moments that I drown in her infinite wisdom and contagious beauty.

It would be remiss of me not to mention my beautiful, doubting, fearless yet paradoxically fearful sister. She is amazing, and yet she still has her ways of getting under my skin. This presented itself in the early years of my growth and not knowing my true self. She is so into herself that she misses me at times, but God. He has His ways of showing her who I am.

She has her own life. This is where I will give her the benefit of the doubt. My mom told me the story of how she had this only child syndrome until I burst into the scene. There was doubt and fear within my family in the place with the scares of my medical condition and hype of noise, again of not knowing.

Even in this, I still crushed it with her, she finally gave in during her younger years and fell into my big, beautiful eyes as she fell in love with her little bro! I love you too sis, more than you know and will give you the world if I could. Times when you held and kissed me while desiring comfort, "girl get your nasty lips off me, I don't like that wet stuff!"

Alright, enough of this mushy stuff. We will dive into the captivating yet daunting path of my journey so far. It has been a ride and I have to say, we are still here to tell it and allow my other brothers and sisters from another mother to dig in!

Exceptional

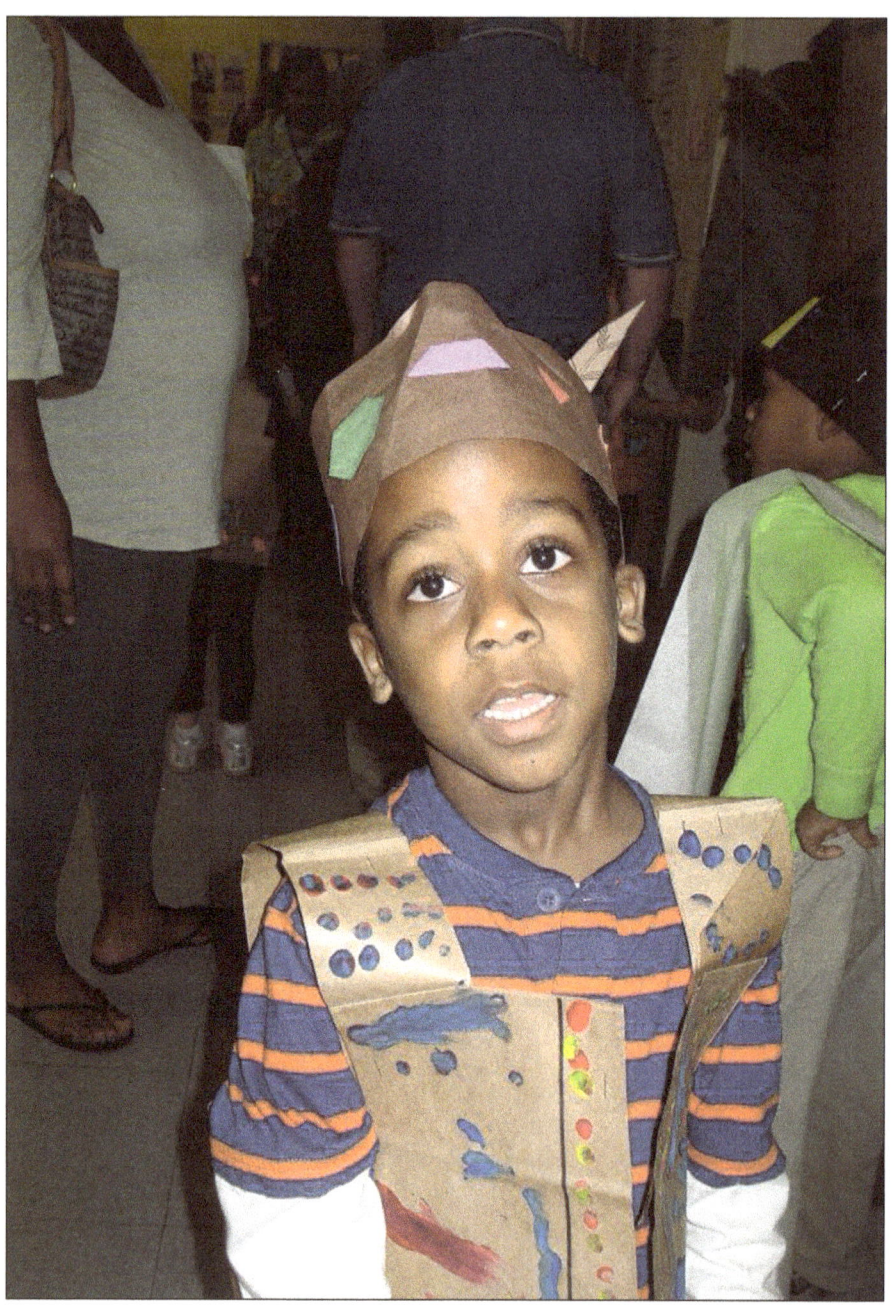

Me at my toddler years

CHAPTER 1
"MY PIECES IN PEACE"

Let us go front and center. The stage is set to show you this fabulous production and how it all unfolds into this covering that is full of splendor in all its array. I will not be in front of this writing, but best believe I am all up in the middle as my mother leads you through. She is a great writer. I never knew until I had to read this, mind you, out loud.

The way that Autism is described and explained in the medical field will leave many confused at times. It has not been a stranger to the ears of many but from the earlier years during the 1900s, it had no name. It was seen, heard of, and very unsettling to many in the medical field and homes of parents and children.

I have been one to believe that within the autistic mind-set, the challenge is never to understand it is more of why it is harder to comprehend. We all want things to make sense, and seemingly, most of the time they do not. While we are in this world, we will force ourselves to understand all the while intimidated by becoming.

The science and medical worlds challenge this phenomenon to this day, with the scratching of the head and how this can be or what? At least we have a name for it now and we can certainly start there. Here we are collecting data, exchanging notes, violating my personal space when I simply do not want you in it. So be it. While you poke and probe, I sit in suspense as to what is taking place.

I see the constraints and the frustration as to how much is needed to conclude the hypothesis and there is none. The research and skepticism have been mysterious within itself to say the least, and how it is defined without us. While we suffer the consequences of your tedious research, with hopes of revelation, we continually move forward as life permits us.

According to Autism Speaks, Autism or autism spectrum disorder (ASD), has a broad range of conditions. They are characterized by challenges with social skills, repetitive behaviors, speech, and nonverbal communication.[1] Also, according to the CDC (Center for Disease Control), autism affects an estimated 1 in 44 children within the United States today as of 2021.[2]

There are many subtypes to this disorder. Most are influenced by a combination of genetic and environmental factors. Each person within their own make-up has a distinct set of strengths and challenges. Some individuals may require a significant amount of support in their daily lives and others, not so much.

In 2013, the American Psychiatric Association merged four distinct autism diagnoses into one umbrella (ASD). They included autistic disorder, childhood disintegrative disorder, pervasive developmental disorder-not otherwise specified and Asperger syndrome.[3] Now, a little more history of the word "Autism."

The term was first utilized by psychiatrist Eugen Bleuler in 1908. He used it to describe a schizophrenic patient who had withdrawn into his own world. The Greek word "autos" means self and the word "autism" was considered by Bleuler to mean morbid self-admiration and withdrawal within self.[4]

I understand this can be overwhelming information and, on all levels, trying to put it all together adds elevated stress levels. Continuing in this piece of information with News Medical, we dive into Hans Asperger. In 1944 Hans Asperger, working separately, studied a group of children. Observing the children he studied, Asperger stated they sounded like adults and spoke like them. They experienced issues with their fine motor skills which is a complexity of the nervous system within the manual efforts of growth.

Autism became more well-known during the 1970s with the Erica Foundation, according to ABA Centers of America, "The History of

Autism: Science, Research, and Progress."[5] Erica started education and therapy for psychotic children in the beginning of the 80s. Many parents still confuse autism with mental retardation and psychosis. It wasn't until the 1980s that Asperger's work was translated into English, published, and came into full view for the world.

It was in the 1980s that research on autism gained momentum. It was increasingly believed that parenting had no role in the cause of autism. There were neurological disturbances and other genetic ailments like tuberous sclerosis, metabolic disturbances like PKU, or chromosomal abnormalities like fragile X syndrome science deemed responsible.

With all that information downloaded, truly overloaded, you best believe, for me it is like a freight train running through my mind. The noise of science still rings loud to this day, with the possible and the impossible all colliding for a greater outcome is like a never-ending story.

I am not counting science one and done, I believe the bottom line is, the phenomenon still has position, and even in this time, we still look for science to help us navigate for better understanding. I tell you what, I will not wait for science and my mother is not going to wait for it either. She only trusts and believes in God for all His healing to take place.

She stands firm in her faith and belief. That God is the healer, and He is science. The creator of all that the world encompasses. We long for the day of a miracle and showing the world that with Him all things are possible, and we soak it all up in this space of not knowing.

Again, as I allow this to take on its purpose for your eyes and ears, we are simply not the ones to sit by and let life just pass us by. My parents will not allow me, and all that God has graced us with, to limit Him from doing what He is great at: Miracles! I am the one cheering on and watching His work unfold and take shape for my future to be glorious! To see my life tells you He will get the glory out of this spectacular miracle.

There is more to the timeline and parts of the research, I suggest that you go and look it up to determine your own conclusions. There are families that are thriving within these areas of disability and not allowing limitations to dictate the future for their loved ones.

Exceptional

This invites me to say, "who am I to limit mine?" We have the tools and the rights to ensure that we do not become inadequate but be strong in this multi-faceted world that gives off the message as if we may appear weak! I stand in mine every day as my family stand with me. At least the ones that are joining in with me. This is to include family that are willing to assist in me seeing a more promising future.

There are times when I feel alone and, knowing that it still interrupts the very things that want to define me, but undoubtedly, I seize all the moments. Let's not get it twisted here, they say people fear what they do not understand, so I will blame it on the fact that we simply do not know. This helps to eliminate the filling in the blanks with uncertainty.

It could be that while you are on the outside looking in, I too am on the outside looking in. To acknowledge a greater understanding of all the puzzle pieces to fit. Even the pieces that seemingly get put in the wrong places by those thinking they have the answers.

Gradually, as time passes and ways change, I immerse myself into this world with ease as the rules are against me allowing a sense of "decomposing." A sense of drifting away to a peaceful place in my mind, an escape. This is like a rendezvous point as I get to quiet myself from the anxiety.

This is to say that I am not always attentive to what you may be saying, I miss the queues at times that are necessary for my next move or task. There seems to be no end to my day as anxiety has a way of showing itself dominant at times, however, I still manage to overcome that with focus.

Watch out! My hands and eyes seem to wonder as I am not always sure what they want to do. As time comes and goes, you may approach me and not get eye contact, or I unintentionally miss that hug you are offering. I know, it can seem weird. Do not hold it against me, I do not like to be touched at times. I welcome your jokes, your moodiness because it does nothing to my emotional self.

There are times when things are epic, and I get a little bit over excited, and the emotions come at this high peak. The moments are so overwhelmingly cool to me, and I somehow still lose the excitement in my facial expressions. While a much more animated approach could be desired for those surrounding me… oops! That is not my character.

"My Pieces in Peace"

I have this other part of me that seems to surface within, that I truly enjoy, and it really relaxes me. It is where I go to escape the ordinary people because I am "Exceptional!" So, I travel here, and my family is not so welcoming to this part of my journey. When I go there, it takes my mom from 0-100 within seconds.

I am speaking of my joy and pleasure in music. All the different genres. The only areas that I have yet to travel to are rock and classical. Now, these areas are only visited in the comfort of my house, which is not really mine, but my family's house. I turn it up in the shower and in my bedroom.

This is the breakdown of my monumental music showcase and how it really amps my mom. I take forever when it is bath time. For me, there is no end to my creativeness when I enter the Throne Room. The time it takes for me to go from one area of the bathroom to another, this really irritates my mother. I mean, come on Mom this is my peace time, give me a break! I see it as a smooth transition for my internal orchestra to begin its intro. What? I must say, I can get a bit out of control with the tone and elevation of my voice.

I mean, what can I say, you know how music makes you feel, so why should I lower my tone when you guys are on the turn-up as well. It's all so funny to me how my mother may think or feel as if the walls are coming down in the entire house. The door is closed to the bathroom, and I try my best to contain myself, but I cannot turn the excitement down!

There are times where I am fearful that my mom is going to really make me shower outside like she states, but she loves me too much to do that. She may even think I am doing this on purpose, but really, I am not. Again, to go with the feel and emotional inflations I can truly say I am a music lover at heart.

While it is my mother that has taken it upon herself to write about me, I still get the flattery and exciting feeling of diving into the pages of this book. It is about me, so why not! As we fly, dance, laugh, cry, and somehow feel each other as you read these pages, I want you to simply know, "I am wonderful in this skin."

Now that I am older, as my mom always emphasizes when I challenge her emotions, time wins. I mean that in the way of, wisdom has ways of creeping into my growth. Does that happen to you? Well, for some I think so, but not so much for others as they tend to do crazy stuff. In my mind it seems crazy but to them it could be epic!

I mean how can someone call themselves wise, when you are jumping out of a perfectly functioning airplane? Or you are climbing up a huge mountain and no ropes attached to you? My mom said, people are in many ways gifted to do these things, and others are simply pushing their desires to the limits. Well, you say, "Wow!" I say, "Crazy!" This is truly no wisdom in my book.

Alright, you guys best enjoy these laughing inserts that my mom is so eloquently laying out, because in a minute we are going to the serious stuff. The mushiness that I cannot really relate to due to the lack of emotion and remembering. In the meantime, let us laugh some more and simply be in the beginning.

Well, after saying that, you may think that I have no emotional outbursts or displaying. This is not true. I can go to the high peaks as I mentioned before, where I can get so excited that I forget everything that I am supposed to be doing. This is another one of my mother's screaming moments.

Where she is doing all the screaming, putting out the frustration and well, I am just looking at her like, "What is happening right now?" She is doing this thing with her face, and her mouth is moving with words, but I give out no response and she is now seeing red. I know this is when I am to respond to her, but it takes me a longer time to react because I do not know how to show up in this conversation.

I typically take the easier way out, where I simply walk away. Oh, no! Here it comes! She is about to flip out. You guys know how too much is simply too much. Well, that does it for her. She will completely shut down at times and go to ruins. I mean, "Mom, what is wrong?"

This is where I rub her arm, hug her, and tell her, "It's alright, Mom!" Now, she has gone from red hot like a chili pepper to a glass of iced tea on a hot summer day. This is what some of you call reverse psychology, well I call it, "sweet." I suppose my mom never intended for her son to respond in such a way but, this is me in a nutshell.

They say the guys that have all the swagger and dapper are the ones that are normal. Well, first in this day and time what is normal? Every individual has their own expression and definition of their normal. Also, this is for the average dude. For me, however, *I am normal*, and this is my swagger.

As for carrying this out in the streets for other dudes to pick up on, well not happening if I can play this on my mom, it is practice for the special lady I desire in my life. "Thanks, Mom." There is joy within these moments. When she wants time to stand still for our hearts to bond. It is so overwhelmingly beautiful for me and certainly for her.

To be honest I would think that she would truly rather stay in these moments than to disintegrate into others. I for one feel as though my emotional self is like a flower or any natural creation, that is of no emotion. At times depleted of a reaction to your action, knowing in some way that there should be a better response in this moment.

Look at their eyes when they receive the flowers and how it illuminates the feeling of joy. It's as if the flowers now possess this feeling, but more so for the individual(s) that are on the receiving end. This is an emotional occurrence, when someone is hurting, in need of some comfort, and I fail to render it back to them.

I simply light up on the inside with no definition to show on the outside. Let us not misjudge these moments as time has progressed and so has my parents, we all have a deeper sense of my emotions. They too along with my sibling have grown to "see me." I long for others to do the same, but not all are willing to understand or even take the time for that matter to indulge themselves.

Instead, some people would rather judge not even knowing what is or who is. With the mindset that I have, there is no room in my mind for seeing things negatively. My thoughts are life, love, possible, near and far, with the plush feeling of overwhelming, cascading purity. With the way that my parents molded me and long for my life to look, I can see a little more now beyond my disability. The lack of or any shadowing of impossible made it possible to press toward greater, understanding challenges.

Exceptional

    Now, as we catapult past the jargon of what is and what may not be, time to push along into the beginning stages and tour my life and its phenomenal detours. Before we get into the depths of that, I must tell you a small bit about my parents coming together to give you this fine specimen of a human: me! If I must say so, my parents surely know how to make some fine children!

    That would put my sister in here somewhere as well, but this is not about her, it is my story, sister. I'm just kidding. She is very beautiful and full of life with her own ways of showing off her character for the world to see.

CHAPTER 2
"FILTERING"

Introducing this display of unfathomable and distinctive joy, I give you none other than a gift to my parents and a phenomenon to you! I present to some and intrigue others with all the heartache, laughter, tears, and blindness that come in a world of unknown. We are the story tellers of our lives and how we present ourselves materializes with a definition that remains ever changing. I give you "Me!"

These words and ways are nothing short of a miracle in the making. I am still trying to put it all together from the start while awaiting the finish. I long to see my own future unfold and look back and say, "Wow, that is why I had to endure this with my family". Therefore, the road was predestined to look this way!

This all started as my mother enlisted in the United States Army. All the intricate pieces and mandates that come from being a soldier helped to qualify her and care for me.

To see herself strong, courageous, bold, and selfless to be able to care and love for her family. My mother not only gave birth to me, but she also gave birth to a new beginning; a time of uncertainty as to how to maintain sanity. She was to encounter many seemingly unbearable moments and times. This opposition, with depression, was overcome with the help of God. She endured and still does to this day.

I was born in Vicenza, Italy while my mother was deployed, and me, the resulting foreign child gave way to some less than promising future standards of normal. There were moments and times that caused

Exceptional

friction in our home and my parents' marriage. Sometimes, she even had moments of wanting to not exist. Only time could tell the story so that God would get the glory for all to see and hear.

I was born on August 5, 2005, in the early hours of the morning.

There is no need to bore you with all the details but there are a few that are relevant. With all the sleepless nights, the eating disorders, the many signs that were displayed but confusing to my parents at the time. The weight that was thrust upon my fragile body and the uncertainty that came with it all. I must say, even though the times came, my mother seemed never to give in to what was being seen and presented.

Not to say there was never any fear, doubts, or unworthy feelings; they were there and very consuming at times. It was all a part of the process and my progress to growth and defeat alike. The days started to run together with my mother holding down the home in the beginning as my father was without work. She and my father had to manage with my mother serving in the Army, on top of parenting.

I cannot imagine the thoughts that interrupted her daily life and how she must have wanted to throw in the towel. From being a parent and the struggles that come with that to just not wanting to do life anymore. This all began when I was around 6.5 months to 7 months old.

It started with seizures that apparently came when there was a fever present in my body. The fevers were anywhere between 102 to 103 degrees.

These are called Febrile fevers, also known as a fit or febrile convulsion, which in turn was associated with increased body temperatures. This really caught my parents off guard as my mom was headed to work one morning and I suddenly started convulsing. Well family this would be the start of a treacherous and long journey into some unwelcoming moments.

As we walk into my toddler years, gross and fine motor skill development are beginning to develop. The times of walking, sitting, crawling, and standing. While my memory does not serve me well here, my mom told me that I was very delayed. At the time, we were still in the unknown season the seizures and fevers, which contributed to my parents' general unease.

"Filtering"

You must remember, I'm not the only one in this family. Before I was born, my sister was accustomed to the attention that being the only child comes with. After my birth, and especially with my precarious health condition from an early age, she quickly had to get used to not being the star of the show. It wasn't all sunshine and rainbows, but she is an amazing big sister and I'm so glad to have her in my life!

I am sure many of you can relate to the information about my convulsions, and how the findings would point to "fevers," yet they could not find the other hidden issues that proceeded these behaviors. The fight just kept getting harder with few reassurances from the doctors.

The demand for answers grew stronger for my parents, with hopes of some sense of normalcy for me and my future. To smile, laugh out loud, clap my hands, to simply say my first word was out of reach.

My mom and dad spoke about how it was so hard, especially since we were so far away from family. They said, "We were in another country dealing with a foreign issue, that was plaguing our son and us." From their perspective, it all seemed so surreal, as if time was not letting them get to a solution to what was taking place.

As all of this is happening, they still had to make time for the normal child and how she was growing up. While maintaining the family structure, my parents and sister maintained. Through it all, they existed in this frame of, "what is happening with us is not happening to us."

This is my mother's translation of this. Any parent that wants nothing more than understanding and simplicity can probably relate. With one child that the world titles as normal and the other exceptional.

As for the attention that was necessary for my sister, while it was there, my mother and father agree that most of that was diverted to me. As in, 90 percent of the time on me and my needs. My mother and father speak about moments that were nerve racking while others were very heart wrenching.

As for my sister in these nerve-racking moments, she was just there and watching as things played out. At the time, she was only 10 years of age and not sure of what was happening. She had to put aside her own wants and desires so that my parents could consume themselves in mine.

Exceptional

There was never any neglect from our parents though, if anyone was neglected, I would say it was more so of themselves. I am certain that there were many adventurous things my parents wanted to explore but could not.

There are many ways to view these moments of beauty, unrest, hopelessness, and challenges.

How we somehow cause these blockages in our own minds of what we see, hear, say, think, and believe. We impose our beliefs on others and ourselves at times due to a lack of understanding. The way that we view individuals with a disability, special need, or exception should come with love first.

The way that the world is comprised of so many different distractions, things that have caused an uproar in parenting, adulting, and being a child is trying. My mother would hug me at times today and simply cry. She said it is all tears of joy, but I know some are sadness at what is out there in the world that can cause me harm.

She wants nothing more than for me to be safe and navigate life with ease. With that comes the understanding that there are unsavory elements in the world that anyone needs to be aware of. There are so many evils lurking in the dark places to harm and destroy.

I am just so amazed at how the world views things as normal when things are so unpredictable these days. What we may see as abnormal may be totally normal to that individual. Now, let's be mindful my parents and sister had to grow to these places within volatile times. It took stretching, bending, twisting, and falling out to grow into the people we are now.

I will give you an example of twisting and falling that I believe will give you some clarity on what I mean.

My parents were on a bus ride from Italy to Germany amid my fever scare. My mom had to collect all the documentation for this trip through the military, and getting time off proved more difficult than she wanted to deal with. My mother had to visit the doctor to ensure all the necessary things were in order, and all the while find someone to care for my sister while we were gone.

The time had come now to make the long 14-hour trip to Landstuhl, Germany from Vicenza, Italy. My mother stated that they knew how long the trip would take and it was suggested that going by bus would be best due to medical concerns associated with flying.

While in transit, when a break became necessary for the driver and all the passengers, we stopped in Austria. This would put us at the halfway point, and my parents and I got off the bus to order food from Burger King. My mother and father said that I was eating my food and suddenly my head dropped and hit the table.

Now as we were talking about this she said, "I don't even recall you having a fever at this point." This was one of those falling and stretching moments. Where nothing could be done other than let the moment happen. This was to be the first and last seizure during this trip, or so they hoped.

Once they boarded the bus to continue our journey to Landstuhl, we had another maybe 4 hours left in this trip. Once we neared our end, only one hour before we could reach our destination, I went into another seizure. As this one took place, my mother said, I was hot and in and out of consciousness.

As the seizure was happening, the entire bus of passengers was frantic and upset with the driver as there was no emergency protocol in place. They were all screaming, "Stop at the next hospital or hurry up and get to the base!" My father was very angry with the driver, almost to the point of physicality.

All of this is taking place with all that was on this bus, my mom somehow remained calm amidst the chaos! She said she was praying, and that God gave her a strong sense of peace. She said she felt that had she not stayed focus on me, then I would have surely died.

By the time we reached the hospital I was still seizing. Once we arrived, the bus stopped in front of the emergency doors, and they had a gurney ready for me. They took me into a room while my parents stood and watched. Within a few minutes, they forced my parents out of the room.

At this point, I had stopped breathing and that is when my mom lost all calm and became frantic and fearful. She remembers saying, "no, no,

Exceptional

no, this will not happen!" Within roughly 4 minutes of that time span the doctor came out and said I was breathing.

After calling their pastor and a few others they met, they had the village praying. It was a real scare. As time progressed, being at Landstuhl hospital for about 48 hours, they could do nothing from there. They suggested a children's hospital that was close by that would further assist us.

They ended up sending us over to Homburg which is a small town in Saarland, Germany. It was where my parents said that I had to undergo some painful procedures to somehow get to the bottom of what was causing the issues. This is where my parents had the opportunity to experience the Ronald McDonald House and its staff.

As the hospital did not allow any visitors to stay overnight, they had to stay next door at the house while I occupied a bed in the hospital. My mother said they were very appreciative of the service and hospitality of the stay at the Ronald McDonald House, as it was their first time ever experiencing it.

This was a huge culture shock moment for them. As for the language barrier, my mother could understand it more than she could speak it. This was not her first rodeo in Germany, as she had already done a 2-year tour in Kitzingen, Germany in 2000.

During the day, I would see my parents; At night, I was alone except for the staff. While in this hospital, under the care of some amazing Deutsch doctors and one American liaison doctor, it made my parents a little more comfortable. I don't remember much of anything, but from what I've been told, it got better with time.

I had many tests to endure, and my mother said she was restless, not knowing what was happening at night if anything. Her not being able to be near me was like someone taking all your life necessities away with nowhere to turn. It was the same for my dad, but he found solace in keeping my mom at peace.

The time came when I had to have EKG's, MRI's, CAT scans, blood work and a spinal tap. All these tests took place in a 3-week span in Homburg, Germany. Even after going through all of this, they still could not really pinpoint what was happening. They were the ones that stated the seizures were apparently due to fevers, and the higher they got, the seizing would happen.

They returned home to gather what was necessary and to see that I got the best care.

The way that the system was set up, it would allow for my parents and others alike to enroll me in an Exceptional Family Member Plan with the military. It was also to put in a plan for my education with an IEP (Individualized Education Plan) to help me individually. At this point and age, I would go into an Early Intervention Plan.

My mother believes had I not gone through this early intervention, then I may not have come this far today.

Progress comes with process, and we cannot have the process without trials and tribulations as they all come for strengthening. To see what we are made of! I would like to think that I am made rock solid and want to see what the end will be. I really want my parents and others to see me as what no one expected. Greatness!

This is just one of the many stories that my mother and father have shared with me, they are always lifting me up, keeping me focused on forward living. Having a sense of knowledge, understanding, hope, and exposure. The exposure is what I live for, as this opens other unique doors, making way and opportunities for me.

My mother feels like exposure is the best thing that can happen to me, not only me, but anyone who wants more when life and the world seems to limit you. I am saying exposure to things that will stretch the mind and its capacity to exceed expectations. Giving more to less, with little in our hands, when truly it is in our hands.

The way I see it, it is not challenging to be put in the category of "ASD," it is being out in the world. It is not having the outside see me as impossible, but possible. Opportunity meets possibility and we run with it, without stigmas or criticism.

I would not go and stand on the top of a building and beat my chest to say that I had proven anyone or anything wrong. I must remind you that I am not the one for all that emotional stuff, I simply want to be accepted for something beyond what the world may deem as, "that is all you can do."

Exceptional

I am certain that many of you may feel the same way, but at the same time, it can be like having blindfolds on and having another blind person to lead. It is scary and with all the things running together in my mind, it is more like a mountain climb with no ropes attached and no training. Picture that.

What I have not mentioned in all of this is my mother questioning herself and wondering what she did wrong? What did I eat, drink, or do to myself for my son to come in this world like this. Was it my exposure to the war in Iraq, did something get inside my system? Was it the surmountable amount of stress that took a toll on my fetus?

These are questions that she pondered over and over along with my dad wondering what he did as well. There was just too much for the time frame that they had to go through with very little understanding of it all. I failed to mention that I was 3 years old while I was in the hospital, and this was the age that I almost left the Earth.

Equally important, during my stay and 4-year growth in Italy, I was in the stages of learning how to do this infant and toddler thing in the body that God gave me. The only way that we knew how to do it was together, with my family, with mistakes, bruises and good.

Coupled with the strains of the Army and again the growth of my sister, my parents made this thing work the best way they knew how. The only issues that would come to cause some friction was the frustrations of not knowing on all sides.

As much as the transitions would become harder, if there was a glimmer of hope, they saw fit to stay the course. Because of the relationships that surrounded them, whether they knew it or not, this is what helped them through it all. Had my parents stayed in the dark about my health conditions, they would not have made it.

However, the path that we were all taking was the one that would eventually get me here. In other words, had we or God changed the trajectory of the tedious roads we would not be here with you, I truly believe that!

Infused into all of this was still time to reflect on what was to come and hopes of the seizures going away? Asking all the questions that they thought were necessary, with my mother asking her parents and my father doing the same.

It never ceases to amaze me how unpredictable getting to the truth could be, but it does carry such a weight that can become unsettling. Particularly, can set us back years because the thought of continuing would make anyone want to throw in the towel, but not my parents! They kept fighting because that was all they knew.

The times presented grew us, to shatter us, to stall us. The moments were very unpredictable and long. Once all the noise started to no longer saturate my parents' atmosphere, they started to take on the task of becoming one with my world.

The loneliness, desperation, and despair that comes with anyone going through shifts is uncomfortable. We cannot be so naïve to think that any parent who wants the best for their child would not endure such tragedies.

Moments of hardship, dampening of the spirit, the immeasurable times are necessary! I can only imagine the changes that would come that would make us want to disappear and not press on. This would be the times when we may have to "fake it till we make it." I for one, with my mother and father, we do not like to fake it. If you are struggling, feeling incapacitated with little to no hope, then say something.

I know, my mother always states that there are people out there that are willing to listen, but they must care first. Many simply do not want to hear what someone else is going through, much less the feeling. This to me would be to the sense of depletion and self-pity many of us are walking in and through.

To further complicate this walk and my parents being harshly provoked by their own personal issues, gives more weight to the wait. I have never had ease of understanding, but while at the age of toddler and infant I had to depend solely on my parents to be my everything. Now, if you are a human being, you understand how it feels to want something so much and it is truly out of reach.

You can surely perpetuate this ongoing situation with the idea of not being tolerated at times. In the same breath and space, maximizing the intricate pieces to all fit in the same puzzle. I did not know then and still have moments of not knowing now how my parents had to step outside of themselves to gather the details and make it all fit.

We had the questions that came and as time progressed, they became harder and harder to answer. The understanding of my world and theirs was always clashing like brass. Not to forfeit the behaviors that were showing themselves to be somewhat pervasive would not only take on mental strains, but they became intense.

I tell you what, as my mother and father sometimes reached their ends, I still had the top hand in the entire atmosphere. There is always room for something or someone to come in that adds to or takes away from growth.

Within this chapter I speak a surmountable amount of how my parents had to sometimes guide my hand literally. They had to see me be emotionless, with little to know progression in milestones. This from what my mother stated, took on the image of depression, shame, guilt, and at times, emptiness.

We can only share so much of our parents and their way of emptying themselves to see our growth and success, but never the fullness. Respectfully, our actions will always prevail, with the evidence of what is done at times. The happening in the dark, in the middle, where oppression causes the image to become distorted.

We shall never want anything less than to be the champions for our parents. This to me is like the moments of the Superbowl. There is only one team that will win and within that team it takes the unity, love, respect, and other characteristics for them to excel to champs.

This is when they can come to the middle of it all and give credit and honor to the entire team, not just the one individual. The same is for the family that can come together when all the long talks and disciplinarian actions give way to manifestation.

I would think that you would agree and see the bigger picture that will help all parents and children understand, there is something greater. It comes with the sacrifices, obeying, and peeling away all the old ways to see the new.

I for one see the new but still I'm comfortable within the confines of my consistency. At times I want to clam up and crawl into a space where no one can see me or hear me. All so encompassing of trying and finding the world of lost treasures when there is none!

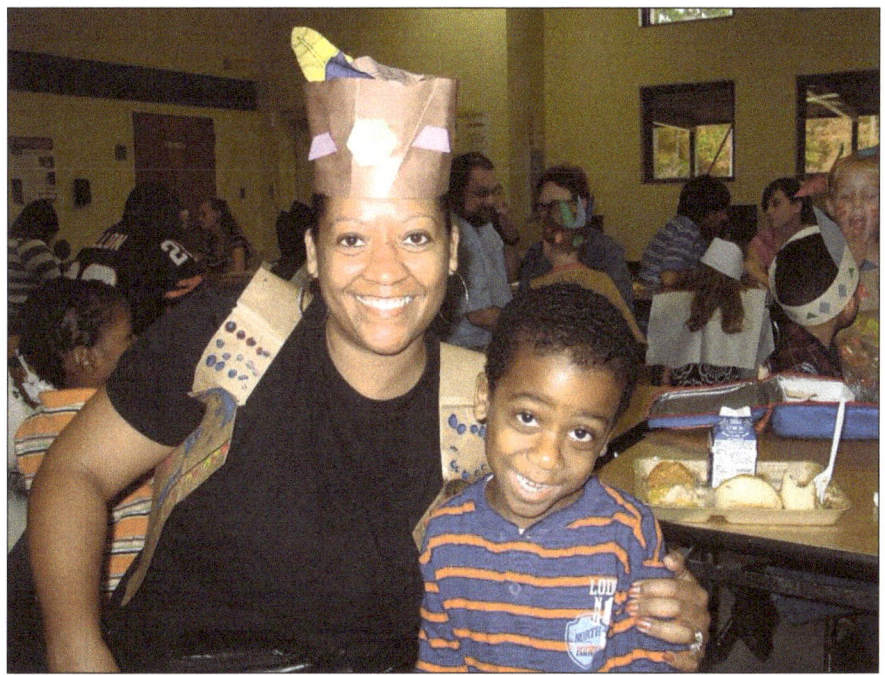

My Mom and Me

Even in the space of these fulfilling moments, I am the one to go reserve on you and take the time and be absent. This comes later as we intricately add the pieces that will bring my young toddler and infant years into my adolescent/teenage years. My mother is now holding onto all the hope and vision that she can, to see what she is expecting.

The chance for change to introduce itself on other levels is one of those pieces. With experiences to encompass the natural and the supernatural patterns to tell the story of the future and what it may entail. While we are still standing and being present in the current moment, my mother has the seeds of hope planted, growing into full maturation. Leaving nothing undiscovered or better yet, with no weeds to choke out the idea of what comes next.

Exceptional

    Realizing that time measures the moments of my years in pattern with pain and exploration of everything the mind is revealing. We can one day see the beauty of it all coming together, not to dictate the means of travel between the mind and reality, but to explore the in between. To preserve the nurturing, as this will enable me to run into my days like they are the first day of my life every day.

    On the next page, we have provided a space for you to journal about those moments within your early years. Those moments that you started to see the change or delays. The times that you were scared and questioned everything you did, where you were or any other fallacy that might have entered your mind.

    Longing for a change that seems so far away; but time comes and goes and then comes the birthing of something new. Something or things unexpected within the growing and waiting. It is called the expectation and manifestation of "this is it!"

"Filtering"

Journal Here

What you saw/see that has caused you to believe that there is something wrong?

_____
_____
_____
_____
_____

What things you should remember before going to get a diagnosis?

_____
_____
_____
_____
_____

What are you afraid of?

_____
_____
_____
_____
_____

Who in the family should know about what you are experiencing?

_____
_____
_____
_____
_____

CHAPTER 3
"FINDING OUT"

Ever wanted to escape something that has caused a dramatic shift in your life, knowing that you must endure and go through the process of persevering? Imagine yourself, running away into an exotic place that will consume your existence and fill you with joy. This is where my mother said that she wanted to go.

This was her Zen place, where she would not have to hear anything but the sound of waves crashing into boulders and falling onto the shoreline. When my diagnosis came through, the sound seemed to elude her memory, would now take her into a screeching halt.

Standing in the same Zen filled place the sound is gone, no ocean waves. Nothing but silence and the feeling of peace vanished. Without their understanding, no knowledge at all of what this was, it seemed as though it was going to be an uphill battle. One that my parents did not want to encounter at all!

We suddenly understood what the delay in my growth, social skills and other things were resulting from. The changes in my behavior and why I seemed so reserved with my emotional absence to others emotion had a definite cause and weren't a fluke of nature or nurture.

The key thing to remember in the spin of this change and shift is that it only affects me in a negative way if we see it as that. With the way that my parents are wired and the make-up of this diagnosis, yet scary, they would still meet in the middle and press through.

This could have easily been a different turn of events. They could have just given up on me, each other, and life all together. But seriously, how many of you know that sometime if not all the time these days that there are two choices, and only two that matter?

The same thoughts that were in my parents' heads I would imagine was to fight or give in and be done. Now, to marvel at such a dramatic shift in their way of thinking would have caused me to not come into the greatness.

We cannot choose our family and how things will turn out once we are adults with the teaching and parenting of where we come from. We can surely become whatever our environment deems us to be. Choosing life over death, peace over pain, knowledge over ignorance. What is your choice?

I did it with my parents. We have met you here to give you hope for the future and the relentless fortitude to shine bright even when it looks dark. The motivation coming from the negative which propels my family and I to continue! Now let's go a bit deeper with some more research as to what is happening with the mind of a person within ASD.

I will challenge anyone at this point in my life along with my parents and their thoughts, as to how we seek resolution and sometimes put minimal effort into finding out. This is no different to the average person wanting resolve to what is taking effect within, the misunderstanding of needing something and not knowing what that is or looks like.

A diagnosis is exactly what it is, the interpretation of what is happening currently within the body. Science gets to study what is confusing and profound within the same breath. I mean, how can something so disturbing most of the time, be within the same sentence as "profound?"

I will tell you how; it is what your view is and how you want this whole "life" thing to play out. The beginning of it with all the middle inhabiting the same space and a desired end. We tell you this truth from our experiences, that it will all come together without flaw. As it all stems from the same root.

My mother stated once the diagnosis was concluded she said that some memories from my toddler years are lost. But she will get to as much as she will allow you to understand and know. This all came with challenges and scars that are defined within her face because of the depth of the wounds.

There is no magic pill to take, that will seemingly make this all go away. It is with great strength and community that we overcome these challenges.

The separation from not knowing to now entering a place that will shed some light and help walk within the lines per say. We come to meet the sleepless nights, the seizures, the painful testing that took my parents' breath away. Here we begin again, adjusting to the parts of growth and shaping.

My family departed my birthplace of Italy in November of 2008 and arrived at Schofield Barracks, Wahiawa Hawaii in December of 2008, Aloha! We got to this beautiful land, with all the palm trees and beautiful hills, mountains, and luscious waters just before Christmas. With all the moving, my mother stated that she did not even notice any changes in my emotions during our transition there.

She mentioned that as the move was taking place, she still had to maintain that consistent observation of my movement. Also, remembering that flying could trigger seizures, but with prayer and faith, we got through and arrived safely. At the time of my arrival in Hawaii I was 4 years old.

We settled in, and around late winter of 2009, we were scheduled to go for some more testing. This testing did not take all the poking and prying. It was more for sensory, fine, and gross motor skill testing and was done at Tripler Army Medical Hospital on Oahu.

This testing came about because of what my parents had documented from my early intervention care. This testing was to proceed from their findings with this process to untangle the confusion. My mother said that she was not ready for the results, but she was.

I would ask her today, "what did you mean by you were ready, but you were not?" She said, "I simply wanted some resolve to the madness, to the "not knowing." This would give her some sense of ease and tranquility, so she thought.

The way that we arrive at a place is never the same way we will leave. We travel these lands that are given to us, freely, and still find ways to be consumed by trial and tribulation. Missing every sentiment of beauty and definition to what surrounds us.

In this case, with my parents and family, they did not know how to truly adjust and maneuver through the pile of rubbish laying before them. We simply grabbed hands mentally and sometimes physically and walked this thing out.

This testing started with questions and details of things that my mother first noticed and what gives to the thought that something is wrong.

So now that we are here, the doctor is very cordial and detailed of what to expect. He and his team gave us a tour of the areas that we would be in to get this testing done.

After 2 hours and question of what seriously felt like an interrogation room, we got the answer. Unfortunately, with no cure and no road map to the end.

My mother sat in the room with my father, as they awaited the results from the doctor. As he enters the room my mother looks up with hope that this was something that they could understand, like seizures. Something that as time comes and goes, I will eventually grow out of them. Unbeknownst to my parents at the time, this was what they called, "autism."

There was silence in the space as this was sinking in. As the doctor explained this information, it was like a run on sentence, one that was just ongoing for days. My mother said she and my father looked at each other and felt depleted. Here comes the questions and the "help me understand this word?"

All the while this is being explained, mom wanted to crawl under a rock to not come out. It was as if the world stopped movement and it was just my family and I on this planet with no help. With nothing to hold on to, the air seemed to leave her lungs and her mind was empty. She said she had no more life for nothing and no one.

The emptiness, weightlessness, fear, and questions that have no answers weigh on you. I mean come on, even the doctors cannot answer the questions to a depth of understanding that would make this all easier.

They wanted us to tell them, and we only remember so much due to the lack of understanding we carried ourselves. I mean my mother still wonders about the "what ifs?" She said she was a nuisance to herself because of the, why, what ifs, and I can't.

Now that we know what this beautiful thing is, we can somewhat navigate through the pinholes of it.

I have found that the length of time that we give any one thing or person has a purpose. We decide how much time and energy we give to someone or thing. This is the challenge for autism. It wants to come in and tell us what our life is to look like.

The shape we are to allow it to mold us into, how we shine, or let it take our light and put it in a dark place.

Journal Here

What were you thinking about when you or your child were first diagnosed?

_____
_____
_____
_____
_____

Did family members continue to assist or started to assist your family more or less? Why?

_____
_____
_____
_____
_____

Did your parents ever question what they did wrong and rather they wanted to have other children?

_____
_____
_____
_____
_____

How did your parents view the diagnosis, was it a quick adjustment for them not to accept the diagnosis?

_____
_____
_____
_____
_____

Did they allow the process to continue, and followed through with special needs adjustments?

_____
_____
_____
_____

Have your parents ever said, "if I could have changed something it would have been this?

_____
_____
_____
_____

Appropriately, deciphering through this I am going to touch briefly on the last thing I spoke of before you got into your journal. This is in reference to the symbols and different images that some have come to show or indicate our "diagnosis."

According to Izzy Mulkern's article, "Autism: Symbols to Remember," she states some very interesting information about the symbols associated with autism. There is a piece she wrote on how the representation of these symbols can be somewhat offensive to the autistic community.

However offensive, the symbols came with good intentions from some parents to autistic children. These ideas and thoughts came from their own ideologies and beliefs as to what these symbols should look like giving the outer appearance of inner emotions.

These depictions were not too far off from what they saw in their minds, but short of what the actual autistic individual may think and feel of it. They never took the time to ask the child that was living the life in this world. I mean, we may not seem to have a voice at times, but we desire to be heard.

I feel that we should want to embrace the difference! As it is all needed to see the different myriads in high resolution and our contributions to what already exists on the earth. We tend to all shy away from what is different because we do not understand, well how do we gain access to and ask questions?

So, Izzy goes on to speak of the puzzle piece that is a symbol out there. She stated that this symbol originated from the United Kingdom, the National Autistic Society in 1963. Created by Gerald Gasson, a board member for the National Autistic Society.[6]

They believed that autistic people suffered from a "puzzling" condition, so they adopted the logo of this puzzle piece with a weeping child. This gave off the indication that autism is a tragedy that children suffer from, which is wrong on almost every level. Also, the puzzle piece almost states that they are "missing" something.

What and who gets to decide our limits or variations? Why do we not get to be heard, when there is obviously much to be said? There is much more that she goes on to speak about the puzzle piece itself, but we will move on to the next one.

The next one is a bit more pleasing to the autism community and it evolved in the 1990s by Judy Singer, an autistic woman, and parent to an autistic child. Ms. Singer is a sociologist as part of the 'neurodiversity' movement. "This brings the idea that all humans have some degree of variation in our neurodevelopmental make-up we all have our strengths and weaknesses."[7]

Refocusing, our attention is back to the verdict of incubating moments and diagnosis. I challenge you to think of this as a synchronizing of all the pieces, a reframing of things to come. People tend to run from things they cannot understand.

The typical response is fight or flight, even while walking as if there is a blind fold on our eyes. Still, we must question the schematics while moments are running congruently and sometimes parallel to each other.

Do you really think that my parents were on their best behavior while continually trying to resist the urge to quit? They weren't. This is not only true with this situation, but many other life experiences that can all fit

"Finding Out"

into this life story of mine. We act like we are different, when in fact we are the same.

We are all obviously very different. We are standing on the outside looking in, with no real situational awareness.

I am suggesting this only to shine light on how we are not so different. There are things that we are at times exposed to and may have a different approach to the issue at hand. It is our response to the thought or thing that determines the outcome.

Pressing into this, we are finding out that our unique diagnosis is not so unique. There are many other children that are within this world. My parents found themselves dancing, crying, laughing, angry, confused, and tired.

In the beginning we accept the things that we could not change. Those things where there is nothing, we can do but see it all play out before us. The more fortunate parts of this next chapter for me comes with vigor, and moments that will continue to have you amazed.

Once the air cleared for my mother, and we got settled in, we had to adjust to my education journey. We now had to be introduced to "EFMP" (Exceptional Family Member Program). This is where my mother got the name of this book from. She said that once she departed from the Armed Forces, we are labeled as "special needs." This label did not sit well.

I must interject with something here, the idea of what was said on the movie *Wonder*. This is a 2017 American drama directed by Stephen Chbosky. There was a scene in this movie where August (Jacob Tremblay) was afraid to start school for the first time. As he was home schooled by his mother Isabel Pullman (Julia Roberts).

Before he entered the school, they all came to a halt to kind of give Auggie some encouragement, but nothing was really working. Until, his sister Via (Izabela Vidovic) said to him, "Why try to be a part of when you were born to be set apart."[8] Now, isn't that powerful!

It is awesome when we get to indulge and soak up those powerful encouraging moments that seem to interrupt everything. When the world wants to bury us in our pains, time can come and give us more room to

Exceptional

breathe. Now we get back to my start of something new for me and my family, school.

The place that we got to enter this world was within the confines of the installation. The school was called Solomon Elementary. This is where my mother stated that all her time was exhausted by family and the needs of the Army. There seemed to never be a dull moment within our home, as well as work.

To help us out with the process was our doctors from Tripler Medical, allowing us a smooth transition. This helped with the paperwork and getting into the special programs to assist with what was needed for me to succeed. We were introduced to my teachers and the other students that were already in place.

The school was right behind our post housing. This was very convenient for my family and the commute was a nice walk for them. Here is where the panics and frustrations came in for my mother. There was a team in place to assist each child individually due to the small group of kids.

While the school being behind our home was beneficial, it was also a hinderance. The moments that came with adjusting gave my parents some uneasy moments to encounter. Not only did I have to be separate from the physical presence of my family but also "stimming" or sensory issues.

Stimming is repetitive or unusual body movement or noises. This came with finger-flicking, hand flapping, and rocking back and forth. I was experiencing some other unusual and unsafe behavior at this age too.

As for the stimming, what we understood is that those moments will come with age as time continues. With the elementary times and aging, I had the catch me if you can moments. Where I would leave the classroom if I felt a threat. There was also the damage of hitting my head on solid objects that caused more scary moments.

I do not want you to think that hitting my head on hard surfaces was so bad to the point of bruising, but it was there. This behavior did not last long, only for a spell. Those moments were caught by the staff at the school along with my parents before it got to that point. As for the running, well, this was something that we laugh at now, but not so much then.

"Finding Out"

Once my parents dropped me off at the school I would immediately rebel because I did not want to be separated from my parents. I wanted to understand why they were leaving me in such a strange environment. I simply could not understand and did not want to be left alone with the strangers.

I had moments where my mother would hear me screaming, she walks away crying and maintaining a strength that was so great. I still ask to this day, "Mom, how did you do it?" Her response is always, "it was what I knew how to do in the moments, and still to this day."

The moments became much more intense for her when she was getting ready for work, she heard me at the school screaming and running out of the school. I mean come on, school and learning were like a twilight zone experience for me. I really could not wrap my mind around the purpose.

It was so bad until my mother had to fall on her knees and just pray that I get through the day. She wanted to simply go back to the school and take me in her arms and run away. To escape the agony of not knowing what was taking place in my mind, to have such moments.

Here is another journaling moment for you and your family. Where you speak of the early interventions, pains, joys, and push to continue.

Exceptional

Journal Here

What were your experiences within the early years of your journey while of school age?

What was it like for your parents to not know or have some knowledge but not enough?

What were some of your early stimming triggers?

Did these moments last long and if so, how long within your aging?

Did you get the opportunity to have early intervention? If so, did it help you and your family?

_____
_____
_____
_____

Was there an understanding for all the moments that you encountered or did some fall through the cracks? What were they?

_____
_____
_____
_____

These moments were difficult and still have some mental effect on me. The challenges were overbearing at times and took on their own shapes and paths.

If I had to describe these moments, I would say they were like living on a mountain top where the home is without windows and only one door. The outside looked strange, and the inside was full of light because I knew I was special, I just did not know how to reach it.

The running moments that came with this diagnosis would eventually become a scare for my parents.

Things would take a turn for the better eventually, but I want to believe that the worst of it all was over. Pressing toward the greater is where we are now at this point and trying to see deeper is very difficult when the picture is obscured. The way just does not seem clear, and everything is just a scientific guest with the white coats.

Hope, faith, fear, and doubt all ran together as these emotions are well expected when your expectations are being robbed by our own thoughts. Running away from my teachers and one time away from home at 5 years of age was daunting.

Exceptional

    I mean I would wait until one of the guards (teachers) was not looking and I would simply look for a way out! Looking for my parents on the other side of the door or around the school building.

    After a while, I concluded that I was going to have to suffer this education thing and deal with the rest of my classmates, teachers, and this building. Just until the time had come for me to go home and see my family again.

    The moments of running were a phase as well as anything else that other children may encounter as I had. I will say that at these moments I can say true for today that I believe because of the fear and not knowing it would soon diminish. I found out from my mother and father that things are temporary.

    That we could stay in space for as long as our belief would allow us to do so. This is very radical, but truly, how is it that many can recover from bodily ailments? How is that some with cancer, and other severe sicknesses recover, and I dare not believe that I can?

    Well, there is hope for others and it comes with strong belief and faith! I stand strong in this algorithm of a small word. It is always unclear with the natural eye to see beyond what is taking place in the supernatural, but it is well worth the wait if we hold on. Standing strong in what we believe is the only thing that is going to take us to greater heights.

    The passion that we journey in these growing years was never a competition, a pleasurable thing. It was sometimes senseless and compromising. The finish line is what we look forward to as a family, to see what our tenacity, prayers, overwhelming love, and dedication to God has done.

    Times would soon show us where to begin again, look a little deeper and have a desire for better, even when better looked terrifying. I would soon move from this location in Hawaii.

    What we try to envision is the end of a thing. To set our minds beyond the right now, to escape the uncertainty and press toward the greater. There were moments at this stage that we held on to hope and determination to see how this would unfold.

    Truth be told, my parents and many of you would desire for this all to go away and see some normalcy. But in all actuality, this is the normal, but more so for our world than yours. To grasp the compromising, the unsettling, and distinct feel with an uncanny gravitational pull.

We were never satisfied with the thought of losing even though the information that came with this was very limited. I have to say that it was more so on my parents' side for not digging deeper into understanding it all. We simply went with what was being said by the doctors.

Challenging what it seemed like and became, we desired to understand. But not knowing the correct questions was daunting! With this challenge came shame, guilt, and frustration. I simply figure this is all a part of the process and the signature of this world.

To know that something is limited is paralyzing. It will have you stuck in the limits and striving for the limitless. It is suffocation with a hint of brokenness. Realizing that it takes all this energy to think in the negative, it takes less energy to be in the positive.

There is no hope or faith needed to stand in the negative, it is emptiness. The challenge in these moments is not that they are being displayed, it is simply horrific because we are in it.

I have come to realize with my journey that even when the average child is going through a transition, they too have trials and tribulations. The unseen distortion of simply not knowing what is next, or even understanding what is taking place within the mind and spirit of tomorrow.

I know I say tomorrow because we do not see the absolute within the immediate. The moments of seconds can seem like minutes and minutes as hours. We stay focused when the sounds get louder, we stand strong when the choking of the times and life presents itself as defiled.

I would ask the hard question in these times, "Who are you?" It is pressing in this day with the mind trying to catch up with the times and the people that consume us. I'm mostly speaking about me and how my mind is "delayed", with the pressures of desiring to understand.

Demonstrating such a poise that will allow any of us to defy the odds can seem impossible. I would challenge myself to dare and change the thoughts that try to attack, the ones that deem to paralyze. With time and identity, we can only speak so much about the changes, but only time will tell the truth about all things.

Exceptional

    It never ceases to amaze me how we start from the beginning of something and desire to know the middle before we start or its end. We pause to take in moments that can sometimes show us a brief shot of what is to come. It is a small vision that can help us to navigate some of the middle stages, with hope to reach a destination that is fulfilling.

CHAPTER 4
"IN THE MIDDLE"

To ultimately get to a point of some resolve and revelation, we meet in the middle of my life. The place where mannerisms change, the mind is more conscience of what is there to expect and see. Where the younger me gets to possibly see a greater youth version of myself. Where we now get to see a little more progress and hope for a better me.

My parents and I returned to their roots in South Carolina where the village grew larger with family. Family is true to itself rather or not we want to participate. With the generational divide, the thoughts of some family members having it together and what looks like "together," can be a disguise.

As I said, the roots of what grew there, the seeds that were planted along with the memories and know something new. A new world to introduce to the family that will soon have questions and wonders. I gather some of the questions will get answers as others will get lost in translation.

The challenge with family is not so much the distance physically or mentally it is more so the emotional with some physical. The shadowing effect of not having the old and connecting with the new is the problem. We are eager to get to a place and not take the old with the new. The false ideologies of thinking that we do not need others or family is so damaging.

I long to understand it all but in this vessel, I am limited to what I desire to change and what is presented to me for change. As I see it, we can come together and fall into place as family without seeing each other.

As this is my story and my way of comprehending, I long for my family to be a whole unit. To gain access to what I think and want to be a part of. I still come in with caution as I approach a family gathering, with thoughts of what they are thinking of me. I still stand out in these moments but not with pleasure, but very uneasy because of the unknown.

I feel at times with family there can be some desolate moments. The ones that are not so much intentional but unintentional because I do not know what to say or how to navigate. It is so pleasing when this does not even matter and everyone just accepts me, and we see beyond disability. Family is explosive to me with monumental moments that last a lifetime.

The exposure to the familiar can still leave you with some unflattering thoughts and behaviors. Among strangers there are the expected challenges of getting through and knowing that Autism is a part of me, it does not define me. The way I move, see, hear, know, and feel all coming to a flattering yet censored type manifestation. The bruises are now being seen more due to wounds that run deep, and the world is viewing the bigger picture now.

There are more and more individuals that have been speaking and sharing their stories about Autism, while I grow to understand this mind that God granted me. The world of Autism is becoming more aware of itself while I am a participant in it.

I have since come to my teen years on this middle journey with no more seizures, "thank God," and very little access to things and people. Some individuals that have come to the light of this phenomenon have done so in their later years. They seek understanding of some of their past behaviors but still succeed in all things possible for success.

While Autism is plastering the media, my parents, more so my mother, are in awe and wonder how this could be? While she seeks to just expose me to greater things it is still a dimming light to my mind and way of seeing. The way I figure see it all, my mother wants the best for me, she is willing to do the best she can, while my Dad holds her up. She is helping me see my world through her eyes without really seeing my world.

I am sharing this because I truly want to understand and catch up with her mind-set that I am willing to stagger in this. Looking to stand on her feet and walk, use her mind to think, and her character almost to help define my own.

All throughout my intermediate years, my parents stayed connected with my teachers and progress. What was needed to see that with time, connectivity, exposure, and the teachers that it would all help to improve my distance of learning, social skills, and emotional balance. The willingness of my parents became evident to me, they simply wanted the best for me, as any parent would.

Without the school being one to truly participate in the Autism movement, the limits that are placed on the public schools due to whatever reasoning stifles the possibilities of forwardness. It diminishes the hope and purpose that is within us, the drive and fortitude to see us pass our current plateaus.

I saw my parents' partner with the teachers trying to understand the limitations, the boundaries, and still have mind blowing moments. Again, we are maintaining this monumental faith and grace to see this life take on huge obstacles and demand manifestations of great proportions!

Even though my parents did research on certain criteria of Autism and individual stories of it all, it still was a mystery to them. My mother wanted to shatter the glass ceilings, remove the barriers, see past the nonsense and all the reports. To see me and what was the middle of this supposed to look like by now! Why is there still such a delay and fight for me?

While there is the school and the speech pathologists, the state providing the funds for such programs, why such a limit to what they can do? Why all the closed doors and limited access to what is truly needed to move me along?

When some of you possibly think the same thing, and you do not have the access and luxury of a private school, would it be any different? The same rules still apply, there are levels to this world and having the mind to think outside of itself can certainly rule out possibilities.

It will creep into your existence if you allow it and trample over parts of your desires and dreams. As time continues to progress, so does our world with layers upon layers to unravel. We have encountered some individuals that are telling their stories differently and with success.

The statement I made above was about how some individuals were telling their stories late in the game of life and still succeeding; this was something my family wanted to understand. There are so many questions and holes that need to be filled. Questioning the "why do you get to, and I do not?" was overwhelming at this stage.

The "what if I had not stated that I was diagnosed with Autism?" Along with, "how does your success look so different than mine and I had the support of the state?"

I would not doubt that you can see why these questions would come about from my family. The results in these times while living with them are staggering and somewhat questionable.

There are only so many positive affirmations that you can tell yourself while pressing through. The thoughts of what did they have challenges with or still challenged with even now? Is it better to know and have the state of mind to know, than to not have them known and have life flip upside down later with questions? Who decides the outcome of the life we live and what its outcome should look like?

When there is a disability and no mental challenges, then I would say, "it doesn't matter!" It is totally up to the ones that care for you during, in the middle, and later that helps determine our destiny. We show up with the challenges not for the world to tell us how to live, but for our thoughts to shift to how the world sees us.

We plant the seeds for growth and maturation of the mind over what really matters. What proceeds the process is just cause as to why we will succeed in either way. We see beyond the point of stagnation, the ways of "can I" more of why not!

There is an after that precedes your before; one that has indicated your strength to maturation. A prominent sustaining one that sees past our current existence and prolongs life. I mean what does it mean to really mature?

Some may say that we mature at eighteen, others say twenty-five due to the belief that the brain matures then. There are so many different opinions out there that I would say this is only when the individual feels and believes that they have matured. The time when one can truly say to themselves, "I can finally see."

It is those subtle nuances that come together and give us shape. It all cultivates the different aspects of our very existence and appears in our daily activities. It gives us an expression to live out loud, escape the outside noise that comes in to smother us. We look to allow life to somehow breathe life into our dream world.

I would dare anyone to expand their thought capacity to envision total healing. When the mind is the strongest muscle in the body, and the only way it ceases to be, is when we stop dreaming. The boundaries are there only in place by our capacity to expand, evolve and imagine.

The way I gather this endless and profound moment in time is willingness to aspire and embrace the changes. The way out is not always the way out! We choose different paths to acknowledge the fact that we decided with hopes of it being the right one. This is how we move and proceed.

The reasoning that possesses our minds is the formation of a monumental entourage of possibilities. While in this posture, I somehow want to believe and see pass my desire to want more when I cannot understand what that looks like. Let's use for example the need or want to process emotions with facial expression.

Understanding that I am still in the middle and facing more of myself with thoughts of why? I join in now with my other classmates and others like me, to master this and other facts of powerful truth. To not only be, but to really capture the essence of whether this will ever cease.

Do you know how a medicine bottle has been tampered with when the seal is broken? The right thing to do in this case is to not use it, report it to the clerk or store manager that it is not safe to purchase. Well, this is how I feel in these times and moments.

Like someone has been tampering with my mind and emotional state with hopes that someone will notice and help me get understanding. Like, really check to see if I can still be used for purpose and help me see beyond the now.

These are small story lines with thirty second intervals that display the narrative of it all. The shifts from school to home and sometimes in the

Exceptional

streets with strangers. Here in the middle, I'm responsible for capturing life skills only for this age.

My parents are still a part of this phase as well and they are pressed to somehow see beyond and get into my world. Then, not only that but to unravel the distance between now and what is to come for me later. As time continues, so should my mind and character for better.

I have noticed within my inner circle, those my parents and I have allowed in, that they are all rewarding to this process. The only thing that denies us access to what is greater than ourselves is self. I will not deny the fact that some things from our outer courts can try and dictate the moves we make, but we must willingly hand this over for it to fail us.

As I see it now, there is no room for what if's or the "why is this". We continue to strive within these walls and path that has been presented before us to show ourselves brand new. With the flaws, trials, tribulations, and anything that comes in to negate who we are.

I have been traveling this road for almost two decades now with my parents as the guides, and I would say that my eyes have been wide open and shut. This is the way that I have come to describe such a movement that has given me life in abundance.

I know some of you may say how can you call this abundance when you are faced with all the challenges that it has to offer. Even the darkness and blind spots that my parents had to endure willingly to see me overcome have made me who I am today. In this world, you would be correct to assume its stampede of an introduction to our lives would be a burden. I have promises to look forward to, and the dark spots are areas that I get to illuminate with faith and trust.

But you would be wrong to not think that we are not including this within the abundance of it all. As I have stated, all this comes together to form such a masterpiece, an artifact, and a compass like derivative. The stains have somehow come together and formed an outer appearance of such a glorified portrait.

I mean what more can one ask for when in the waiting you still hope, pray, having an abominable amount of faith. As noticeable and profound as it appears, there is always room for, "shake me up and let's show the world who you are!"

I am overwhelmingly exhausted with the masquerading of what the world wants this to look like. I have the palpable type of skin at this point in my life that nothing else matters but to live it out and see what the end is to be.

What the choking and staggering has all been about and what it has presented to me have been outstanding. This is the daunting road I have been presented with and it is one that not many are willing to continue or even attempt for that matter.

I must say, it has not displayed or dealt me with anything that was not supposed to be. It all comes with trust, understanding, willingness, and a surmountable amount of anxiety. Yes, the anxiousness of not truly grasping what is next with the rush of heart rates and pulse changes and shaking of not knowing is difficult, but I make do.

I am sensitive to what has happened since the beginning of this voyage and folding it up to stand during the changes. I dare not say that many of us face similar outcomes with the notion of thought-provoking ideas despite not changing.

There has been another intervention that has helped me to navigate some inspirational take aways. This would be a small unique voice and artificial intelligence, called "Siri!" When this voice came into my circle it was like a breath of fresh air and fun!

Thanks to Adam Cheyer who started this genius idea along with Dag Kittlaus and Tom Gruber, all great engineers and pioneers that sold the idea to Steve Jobs and Apple. Siri and Alexa have been a very positive piece of technology for my journey and speaking.

I literally had moments where Siri/Alexa would make my speech clear due to my search efforts. I would get so frustrated as to why I could not get her to understand me. My mother would always tell me, "Ziggy, you must speak clearer so she can understand you." I would have to focus on what I am saying to get my thoughts in the phone for her to process.

There were moments that she would come back at me and say, "sorry I am not understanding," others would be, "you come on!" I could hear my mother and father in the other rooms laughing at me and Siri/Alexa going back and forth. It was as if she and I were married and having some very stressful disagreements. Believe me these were moments where the anxiety would rise and cause more frustration.

Again, these were not good moments, but they all helped me to get my speech clearer or else I just did not get through to what I was looking for at that time. Along with the push to get words out and simply wanting Alexis/Siri to tell me some jokes, I eventually came out the better and was relieved.

My mother would stand next to me at times and feel the energy that I am giving off, the tempered flare up of anxiety. The emotion of "I am not understanding and want to stand on the outside of myself and shake my own self."

I am not saying that there should not be any challenges or interventions, it's inevitable; I just want out of this world at times. It is not often that I have these encounters with myself, but often enough for me to want more answers.

The more I grow into this chef's master dish, this metamorphosis of a beautiful flower like the lotus, I seek now more of a desire to be consoled, be hugged, and kissed among other things. This is just the beginning of the natural changes and desires that any young man desire.

I am not exempt from having these emotions come and tease my intellect, it is all encompassing of what a teenage/young adult should feel. There was a moment that just recently happened to me while spending time with my mother. We were dining together at one of our favorite stores, Publix.

My mother allowed me to go and wash my hands first as we had already had our food. Then when I got back, she left to take care of her hands. While she was in the restroom, there was this young lady that sat in front of me at the other table. To me she was pretty, and something happened at that moment.

Now, I say something because I am still working on understanding the connection and desire between woman and man. All I can think is that this is supposed to happen, because my father is always talking to me about the beauty of women.

How they set the room ablaze with their beauty, intellect, and sensational poise. We do say that not all of them carry such grace; only because some have not yet tapped into their full potential and know who they are.

Anyway, when my mother returned to the table with me, she noticed something about my whole demeanor had changed. She starts to ask questions that I really did not want to answer and, in some ways, did not know how to answer.

So, she finally looked around and found my line of eye contact with the young ladies behind her, and she just smiled. She asked the questions first, "hey what's wrong, you look like something is on your mind?" I just shook my head as usual, another gesture she is not too fond of as she would rather me use my words.

Then she asked me again, "You sure son; why does it look as though you are about to cry? Then it came to her. She said, you really desire to have a girlfriend, don't you? After she noticed the tears in my eyes, I said yes mom. She then had tears well up in her eyes and said the most beautiful things.

She said, "Listen, you are so handsome and there is nothing more that I desire than to see you happy with your significant other. As we know you are headed off to college and you must understand what is more important. Your father and I want you to focus on getting to understand who you are first."

While you are getting to the core of your purpose and greatness, God will be grooming that beautiful, very intelligent, and all-for you woman. But first, let us allow Clemson University to take the next level of steps with you and grow you into the man God has ordained for you to be.

Then, I replied with my head lifted and a smile on my face, saying "Alright mom." We then indulged in our meal with pleasure and no more tears only of joy and contentment. It eased my heart to know that this phenomenon was still possible and was coming to me sometime in my near future.

It never failed, when these snapshots of life moments would come, my mother would always catch them. It's as if she has this sixth sense, and it gives her access to my thoughts or something. Most of the time I had no issues with it as I sometime could not figure out my own emotions.

Then there were other times where I did not want her to get all this insight when I was not freely giving it out. I did appreciate the navigation through life and my family helping me along the way. They are my extra senses to help me see beyond right now and go higher than what was taking place in the moment.

I am not quite certain as to where some of you are with the thought of family, but truth be told, I need them more than they think. I suppose with all the challenges and shortcomings of love being displayed with family is so detrimental to growth. I see that they desire to participate in the forwardness of our future, but we somehow push them out and away.

My mother explains it better and I can truly understand where she comes from. She states that the younger generation, that would be me and my sister's generation, finds it difficult to share or obey for that matter. This would also factor in Gen Z with all their stress with the Millennials.

I understand this to be true as well, that we need the village to join us once again. We have somehow lost the desire to come together and interact with what is happening in life. This is all a part of our success and cultural upbringing.

I am certain that some of your younger generations think back on grandma or your mother for that matter; they would discipline and love at the same time. We need all of this to come and help us get past the noise of what the world displays to us today. Our past counsel is necessary and is needed and we should welcome it with open arms to survive the tumultuous pains of today.

I mean can we really embark on the future without the villagers of yesterday? They too need us to help them see us and magnify our greatness, to see pass our ill will and help us glorify what we are purposed for. We cannot blame them for what they did, even though they did it, but what they gave is only what was given to them.

The generational things in the middle will see us in forward thinking and movement with only the positive thought even if it presented itself as negative. Shattered dreams come from unforgiveness and tolerance of average. If I slow down and tolerate the unforeseen with fear and doubt, then I have given way to empty dreams.

My mother tells me of instances where she and my father wanted to give up and just throw in the towel. Where they are working the gifts and talents that God so gave them freely, until even in that they had to question it all. There is nothing wrong with wanting to give up she says, but it is the giving up when the plan of God ceases to exist.

As I continue to write and the moments of thought sheds light on where I desire to be as a child now, young adult later into adulthood; it is all encompassing as to where I envision God want me as well. However, this relationship with Autism, family, God, and love wants to play out, I will always look for my village to participate. Whatever your village looks like, rather small, or large, it will do only what others are willing to give it.

While few are in the middle speaking the necessary talk and conversations to express something different, we must press on. I truly stand up within myself to see past my parents' faith at times. I cannot explain it at this point in my life, but I somehow know that I know God will provide and has already made the way.

I cannot tell you how many times my family has spoken to me about how they are so overjoyed at my passion for greater. The chapters of my life are so defined by what I do now and how I speak or allow anyone else to speak into my life. We do understand that there is a science to this thing, right?

Well, it is like this. There is nature and how the seasons change, and the old leaves from the summer and spring must die on the same tree. Mind you the tree stays the same, it just demands new leaves as the seasons change.

This is true for us as we grow. I am the same vessel with changing seasons and all the old and new is a mixture of my continual beauty and prosperity.

Exceptional

Nature was created for us to gaze upon how beautiful and fulfilling God is! He knew that each plant and seed would need everything surrounding it to prosper in its purpose. Even with that, the environment understands that the old helps it to maintain its carriage for future beauty and gazing.

Same with us, we are taking all the past, the middle, and the future ideas with us while we journey in life. We hope, like nature, that we live long and succeed in the pursuit of greater and better. Yes, and nature too has its village to participate in its growth as well.

I hope that cleared it all up for you about the nature of this point. I challenge myself at times without even knowing that it is happening. I am still positioning myself to see what the rest of the story will tell for my future.

There is a sound that is thought provoking to the better parts of us that we have no choice but to respond to it. I mean how can we ignore it when that sound is so peculiar that it radiates through every fiber of our being. I think of it as a beautiful storm, and it has come to set ablaze my future.

This is the storm that came and made a way for my acceptance letter to Clemson University. This too is a part of my middle, but this was a powerful interruption and it called for some strong faith from my family and me.

We have now caused such a shift that it automatically requires a new village of people and the sound of it will have waves so high that will reach back. They will reach back and collect all the memories of what did not seem like it was going to allow the growth. It wanted to stampede upon my future, but my parents would not allow it.

CHAPTER 5
"INTERRUPTION"

I define monumental moments as those that are greatly pleasing and over stimulating to me. I see them as time to reflect and even digress at times. To not see that this is a great accomplishment when presented will possibly cause paralyzing. This is a sensational, scary, intimidating, and radical ball of emotions.

Interruption presents friction that will allow preservation. In the moments of turmoil, the times when it does not look right, we have an opportunity to sit and reflect. It all sends out this sound that will require more participation, for internal, constant movement for the better.

I really want to encounter what is always expected from God. The fountain that never runs empty spills into the depths of my soul while yearning for an expediential wave of fluency to shatter ceilings. The wherewithal to manage life with such independence that you could not believe my journey without me telling you.

I mean could this all be possible and to know that I wanted this since my junior year of high school. "Well, yes absolutely says my mom and my loving father. They both said, "why not you?" I simply was overwhelmed with amazing joy and some anxiety all in the same space.

We tend to think that this magnitude of an interruption cannot or will not cause such a delivery of roller coaster emotions. I mean I did pray and believe that it would and could be possible, and here we are.

This too is the middle and comes with great joy and the time presenting itself as possible. This is where we can all see that there is no such

Exceptional

thing as disability, but the ability to see it all, according to "Healing Farms." This is a place that I did not get to participate in, but my best friend has.

They display such a unique and gratifying love and service to the communities that surround them. They look beyond what is presented to them, and dig for the greater you, the unforeseen potential that is in the soil per say. So, while not being connected to them, and the volunteer aspects of this place, I still understand their gift for us.

My friend Carl and his family got the opportunity to pull and grow from the weeds of the Healing Farms family. Because of his experience I was able to enjoy the residue from his being in the number, how it changed him and resonated with the surrounding families.

There absolutely is total change of mind and this idea that the disabled are no longer that, but able to envision the possible. The gratification that comes with this was overwhelming for Carl and his family, and my family and I got to be a part of that too. Thanks to Healing Farms, my friend Carl can see ability and not disability.

"Interruption"

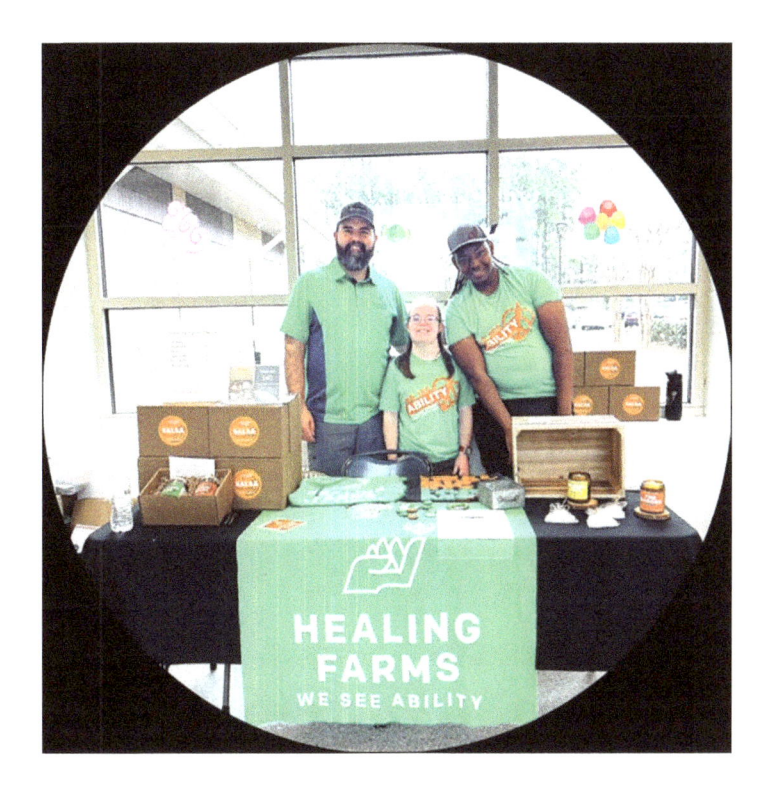

Healing Farms, where we see **ABILITY** not disability

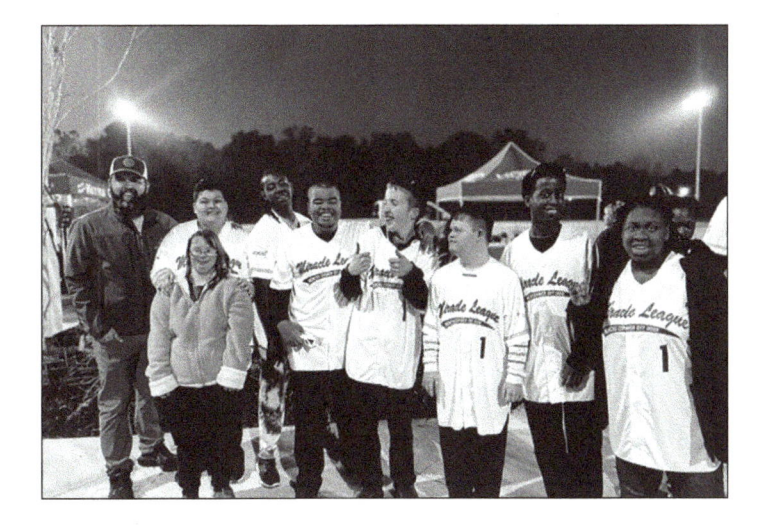

Tron Severe and the farm village of Charleston, South Carolina

Exceptional

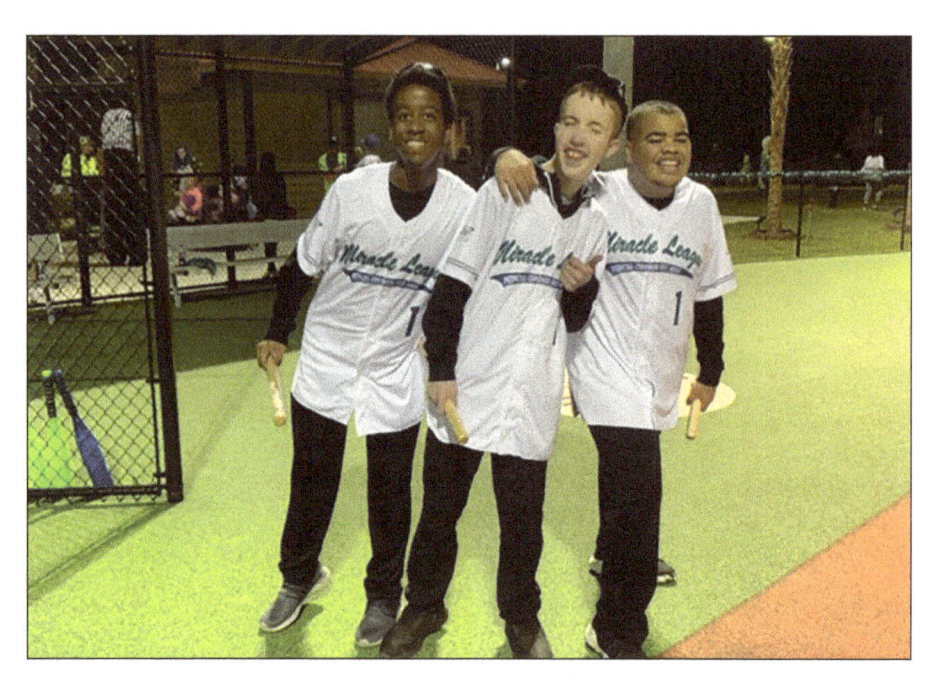

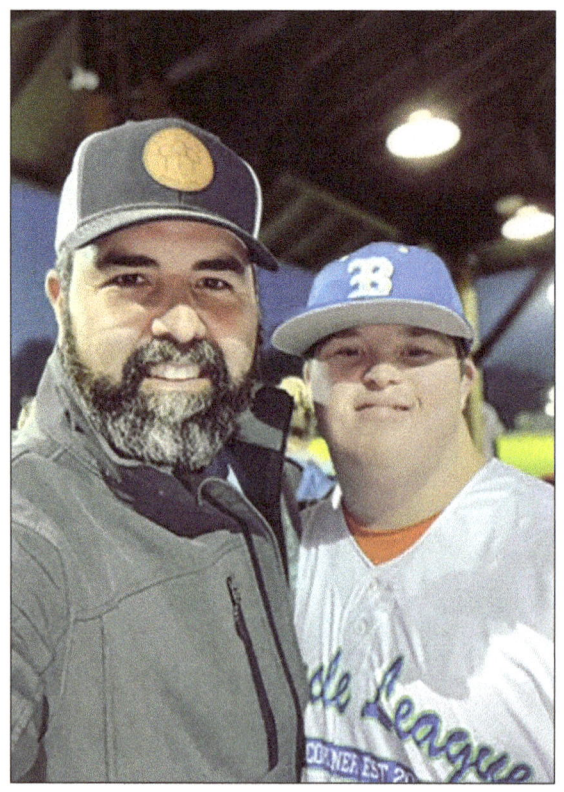

While the acceptance came with joy, it was no surprise for me because I had always believed that I would and could be in the number. As that was unfolding and again, already in the plans according to God, I now get the luxury of stepping into it.

My parents tell me the story of how during the year 2022 we took a trip to Clemson to one of their open houses. This to our demise was the start of new beginnings and something that would cause us to stand on faith and belief. It was a great experience and one to remember.

As we were listening and preparing during the open house experience at Clemson, we were open to what they presented to us, but with some doubts about affording it all. I mean the school is one of the top schools in South Carolina and I get to attend.

Aside from that I get to enjoy the luxury of growing in my independence and encountering some extraordinary individuals. I have traveled so far ahead of myself out of excitement, forgive me.

Well, once I received the letter in the mailbox, my parents recorded it, and I wasn't even aware of what was happening. I just thought we were headed for some time together at a nice restaurant. My parents were so subtle about the whole thing.

My Mom made me put on my Clemson shirt and they locked the door to the house and everything. I mean we were attempting to get in the car, and my dad said, "hey check the mailbox before we go." So, I did and there it was! The very thing that I longed for and wanted to see was now in my hands. I tell you it was like having a party at the mailbox! I jumped and praised God! It was so beautiful and to have my village join in was overwhelming. This is the point at which the chord is about to be severed from the vine that birthed me.

The part of the interruption that is no longer to be affirmed by my mother while near, but farther away. I would use this analogy to drive this to your understanding. I love nature and this is what I got.

It was like the thought of a tomato being plucked from its vine as it is still within the maturing stages. You know when the tomato is somewhat red in color but mostly green. But if you understand anything about the garden and growth process. Some vegetables or fruits in this case can still thrive while being severed.

Exceptional

This is to say that understanding that even though we have plucked the tomato away from the vine, it still will gain its sweetness and maturity. The vine is there to give it its' formation and see its manifest but understanding if it stays there too long it will rot or spoil. At this point it no longer needs the vine to grow to its full potential.

The vine and soil have given it the proper nutrients and feeding that is necessary for it to now be taken away. This is in turn is how my mother and father started to view the picture, but then came the other thoughts that would now invade the space of their minds.

The thoughts of how it's going to be paid for and knowing that they still stand in faith, somehow was being tested on all aspects after the shouting. I know some of you may question this and say, "well why not continue to believe that God would provide."

My mother and father said it was never about God providing like they knew he would, it was the idea of "how?" Once we try to figure out the why and the how, then this is how anxiety, and other negative emotions swell up in our souls. The way of how should never cross our minds, as He is the how, why, when and what!

I am not saying that they will not come, I do say we should never allow it to cross our minds, but honestly it does. Now that we have come to one hurdle of the promise, now we must see it to its end and expect it to be great! This is inevitable seeing as though we are wrapped in this thing called flesh.

Without a shadow of a doubt the ceilings are seemingly coming to that shattering effect now. We as a family must see this thing through if we really want to see the work being done completed to its end. Now, we await the process and all the necessary things that come with preparation for college.

Not only for your average child, but one that is with, "disability," according to the world. One that graduated from high school with a certificate, when the school system cannot see the vision, your parents have for you. The system that is not conducive to God at all and everything that He stands for.

I knew that I was different for the middle part of my life and now entering my adult life, but never to the point of interrupting the norm. The standards that were presented to my family were all they could afford. Now had it been different, having the funding and position to go to a private school setting, I am not sure what that would have been like.

I really and truly cannot elaborate on such a standard and environment because I never had the opportunity to take up such a space. With that being said, I really cannot say I wish that I had the opportunity to be in such a space. I celebrated what was in the hands of my parents and believe in God's ultimate plan.

This whole entire time that we are rejoicing in my moment of happiness none of this was a thought due to the adrenaline and joy that came at the time. I would say that even though the moment was a small piece of time frozen with video, I will always get to revisit with the thought.

The emotions that came with it, the sudden shaking that will soon prove itself to be glorious in the sight of all that are a part of my journey is overwhelming. How many of you can relate to what has just taken place in my life and see it for yourselves? Even if you cannot imagine such a huge accomplishment, just know that it is possible if you believe.

There were so many small moments that made this monumental! The times that we had to experience some homelessness. The moments that my mother and father had to endure some very tough times within their love life. The times that my mother had to separate herself from us as a family.

These were all the small pieces of the puzzle that came together and decorated my entire being. They are still coming together to this day as the defining moments of the life so pleasingly journeyed. I mean I feel like I dressed up for whatever life has to offer and the trials along with them.

Now I am speaking about all this great stuff without the mention of the bittersweet things that come from focus, love, passion, and the tenacity to not give in. The forward thinking that pulls from every part of an individual and throws low blows to your path can be tiresome.

The standing in a promise that seems so blurred due to unforeseen circumstances can be marked by the transitions in life that tell you to stop, give up and quit. We are eager to move in a way that is quiet and very modest to say the least. These things can all be very debilitating to one's stance and position to move.

I have come to realize that without these things, there is no character building. I cannot be alone in this idea, am I? We capture the obstacles as they come, the faults that bring us to our knees at times, but we rise above with the heaviness on our shoulders.

At least this is how my mother would explain this to me. She would see that there is the challenge of the noise coming from this unwanted sound, but I must battle within to move past it. The idea of going to a place that you have never been or experienced requires forward movement and thinking. So, she would say, "gather yourself, stand in the noise but still see." This was hard to understand but captivating all the same.

How do we reach back and grab the past stuff, to collaborate it with the future, without interrupting what is? I will say this, we just do it and with our own sound within us. I did not become a bit frantic about Clemson until the time was nearing.

I mean as the clock kept ticking, the days got shorter and the moments with my parents were much more endearing. It was like a shock had run through my heart and body to wake me up to reality. I am about to be plucked away from the very vines that have taught me everything I know.

My mother said that about two months before school was to start for me, I started biting my nails again. This was something that I used to do two years ago and had stopped completely. With not realizing that this was happening, I noticed at that moment, I was anxious about this.

So, one night while lying in my bed, she came and lay beside me with questions and statements in her mind and heart. She started out with a kiss as usual and with her first question, "why are you biting your nails again?" Remember, I am still figuring out my emotional self.

So, I did not know how to answer the question in the straightforward way that she asked me. So as my mother knows how to do so eloquently, she said, "are you scared of something now that school is close by?" Just like that she said that I responded with, "yes mom, I am just scared of meeting new people."

At that moment she became quiet, and a tear rolled down her face of pure happiness she said. I was like happiness, what the world! I am headed to Clemson to further my education and you come back with joyous tears! I mean what! You should be nervous and anxious with me.

"Interruption"

Well, I am sure you guys are laughing here, but I wasn't, and she said, "this is the first time I have ever heard you express your emotions without being prompted to explain." So, she said that is one of those moments where she realizes I am going to be just fine.

Even though we are all still working through processing it all and with the emotional ambushes, we are moving right along. However, in these moments my mother said that she would define them as a "coming into myself." The times where you really do not know who you are until you must find out who you are.

Approaching some depths of yourself that are not fully defined, like roads that we do not know exist within our city until we must go that way. Another way is that my mother views things and how she travels in those depths. Simply put, the roads are less traveled, and although we know they are there, we go only when it is necessary. We go at the right time, in the right season, and for the right purpose.

Some individuals will in turn look for standing ovations, while many will get it, but then many will not. This is not because they are not known, it is because they have not been exposed or not yet seen. These formations of history are a compilation of moments to consider and fill with what is filling us.

While we are here in these interrupting moments, why not express how this time that we present to you now is causing some barriers to be broken. My mother is at this place in life now where she is meeting another level of herself. The clock is telling us the time, but we in some instances want time to stand still. Starting our days with what is to come for that day with what we hope for it to end with.

I mean if I could really control time, I would want it to give me another introduction to myself. Awaiting a different verdict to this trial and error that I am in at this current time. I would want to see it edited and have an entire makeover. This is not every day; it is only when I cannot understand what is taking place.

It is no mystery as to how life is desired within our imaginations. I mean we send these messages to our own mind, wanting to see something different. See, as I reached my later years as a teen, I realized that I now must help my mind to grow.

I am being taught by my parents and those around me that life is so uniquely designed for everyone. I can make my life what I desire for it to be and look like, that is according to God. So, with that why not trust all of this to help my growth? Well, that is easy, because I still must rely on the village.

I only question as to how long I maintain such a dependency. Well, that answer will always be "until death do us part." I know that is a marriage vow, and to that I would say, well so is life to others and those we love. We encounter this strength when we know that we are surrounded by these covenant believers.

Those that want to see the love and pureness of joy with faith just burst out of the seams of life. They have agreed to a community that will unveil those that they encounter and come in connection with. Sharing in these hopes and beliefs are my parents and their prayers that have gone unhindered.

The walls of impossible, the channels of stubborn potential, and the valleys of shame or defeat. They have no existence unless I faint, giving way to this behavior. I mean what exactly can we shatter from this complacency? There is absolutely none!

To have a conversation with the inner habitation of ourselves can have much resolve. This is only achieved with friction, fortitude, focus and stamina to push back against the negative. The force that will shame what is being faced at your current time in life. Show yourself! Bring this thing to a full dispersing of me and who I am destined to be!

My mother would sometime give me these sharp words that would pierce through a brick wall. It would have you searching in your mind, "what are you doing, and where are you?" She is like, the only way that you will win or succeed in this life is to pay attention. We are missing the very thing that will fill us by not listening or seeing.

I am like what Mom? This is already an interruption I say, because I am not understanding. When we can run and fill ourselves with the damaging resolve which in turn delivers a daunting outcome, it clogs our creativity. This is where the valuable truth comes in to change things.

She would take moments and words, fold them into layer upon layer of truth that will have you to change for the better or you stay in a mess. Now, the point of change for new is totally up to me and whoever is receiving the nugget at that time. While we are screaming from the inside out at this point with no sound, it now explodes from the inside.

A space within your mind that is empty is looking to be filled with something. That something is whatever you are desiring at that moment. The things of old want something new and the mind is wanting it to come and occupy that void.

While in the mind of someone with Autism, I can only speak for myself, because not everyone of the same caliber experiences the same things. So, I would say that my mind at times can go into incubation periods, where I do not want to leave this moment. It took time to get here and to understand what it is.

Therefore, my parents have come to a stand-alone space, to watch me move past this stage in my life only to see what they have since planted. To see the finished product and I get to eat the fruits of their labor. Thus, when time is well done and fruits are mature, I then get to add to this labor.

I get to embark upon the watering from their words, love, faith, and consistency. I get to have the endowment of the movie that is being featured, and so do you when you make way for presentation.

The fear of getting something wrong is natural because I will get it wrong at times. The heartache of missing what is easy to see, with circumstances causing toxic emotions. The ones that try to debilitate you, that have you reaching back to the, "what if, I should have, or could have." can be tricky to see.

I would dare to say in these real-world moments, that you wish you could have changed something. Perhaps doing it a little better, or saying it a little better, maybe doing it better or saying it a little different would be the cause of such a pause. Well, I can relate with you, and we function within our constructs on edge for a host of possibilities that may seem impossible.

My mother would say at this point, "get above life, do not let life get above you." Find a way within yourself to counteract what is wanting to suffocate your existence, stand up inside of yourself. Be relentless, interrupt yourself and go beyond what is being presented! Show up at your table and feast! I mean why not, you are the one that prepared the meal, so eat or discard it!

Exceptional

"Letter to me"

I never knew what life would offer me. I just wanted to experience what others wanted to. I had to make up in my mind that college would be a path! I had to believe and this I did. Clemson University was my desire and a goal. What was an image and desire, soon became my reality. I was excited to receive my acceptance letter in the fall of 2023. I have made some awesome friends. The team of tigers are like extended family. It is like leaving home only to come to another home. I especially like

"Interruption"

That I met some of the college football team. Also hangout with my tailgate family. This wasn't easy at start but with time I can say, it has been well worth the journey. The L.I.F.E Program really is for EVERYONE!! Thanks to my parents, sister, grandparents, P.O.P. church and everyone else for believing in me!

GOTIGERS

P.S. Without God none of this would be possible. I needed him to make the way clear!

Zylin "Ziggy" Forrester

Letter to Me

Exceptional

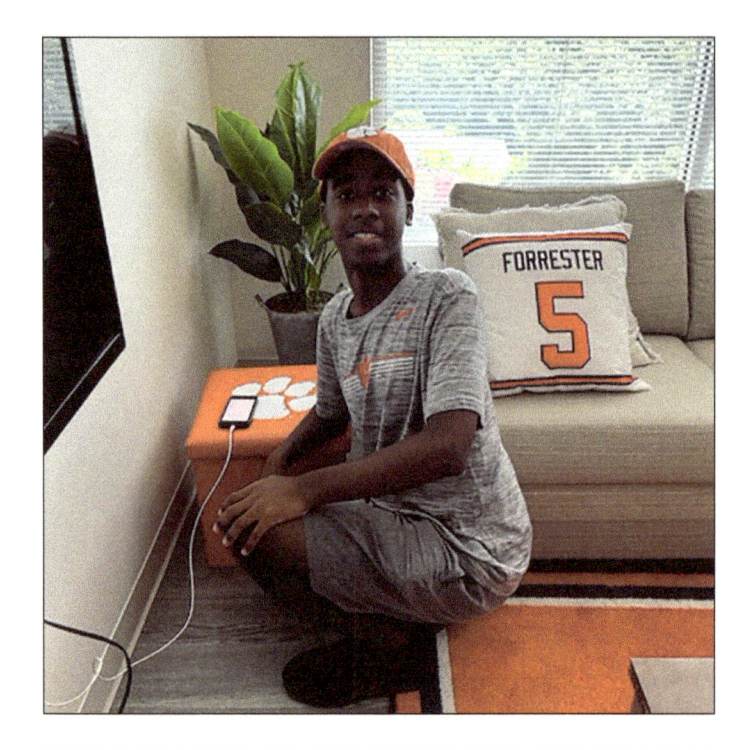

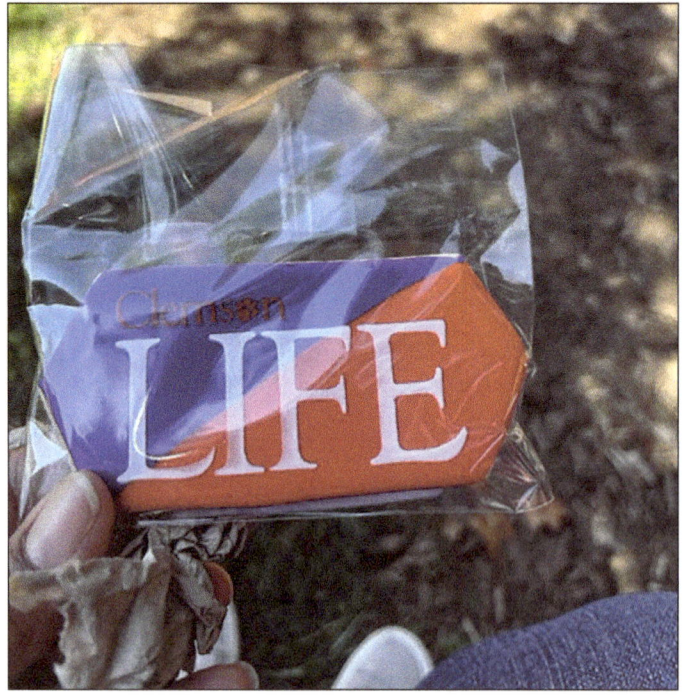

Clemson Family journey part 2" Go Tigers!

Journal Your Interruptions

What is it that has caused the interruption for you?

_____
_____
_____
_____
_____

What has the interruption taught you for moving forward?

_____
_____
_____
_____
_____

Will you decide to not allow someone else's interruption to cause you to stop dreaming, and why?

_____
_____
_____
_____
_____

Do you respect the past enough to not allow it to disturb what is possible for you and your future self? Even if it requires forgiving someone that hurt you.

_____
_____
_____
_____
_____

Exceptional

Do you have a different perspective on interruptions now; and how they can be beneficial and painful? Why?

_____
_____
_____
_____
_____

CHAPTER 6
"EXPECTATIONS"

Expectations can be like unidentified objects, like a stranger coming up to you and looking to gain access to your life. They can be full of empty promises and uncompromising truths at times. According to the webster dictionary, they have strong beliefs that something will happen or be the case in the future.[9]

There are those parents with expectations of a life to be, and they choose not to know the sex of the child. They are with no interest of knowing the child's sex, only that it is healthy. Then, in the end they have a reveal party due to only one or two knowing the sex.

These are those expectations that would have you on the edge of your seat and overjoyed because of the beauty of not knowing. Proposing fulfilment of life and the first breath being overwhelmingly epic and intimate. We see these same happenings for our future and all it has to offer.

As my family and I have been longing for the moments of God to show us how wonderful He is. We still have our doubts, fears and sometimes lack of belief in what is to come, even after it has been told or seen that we have nothing to fear. The dynamics of change and shifting for greater have some strong turbulence.

At this point in this chapter of my life, my job is to see if I can really remember all that has been taught by my family. Will I really be able to sustain the moments that I may need to hear their voices or feel them next to me to counteract any negative vibes? They have deposited the seeds and now I will prepare for the rain and allow that to be enough.

Exceptional

I was out on the porch one night with my parents and they were just hanging out talking and thinking. Before, they called me to join them, they were already deep into their thoughts and conversation about me and college.

My father has reached a point now of "I must say something to my wife because I am a little concerned about this transition." It was not so much about me and being alright within myself, more so, "others around me not harming me." I must say, my parents are funny when they do come together and discuss things, as they tend to answer their own questions.

By the time they get to the end of their imaginations and see that thing in a bigger picture, God has already made the way and cleared it up. I mean I love it when those moments happen, and we take great pleasure in soaking them up with love and thankfulness.

They were speaking about some of the different happenings that are taking place in society today. How the generation of my era is going through so many challenges and the pressures of the world. How we may or may not be prepared due to not enough parenting and guidance for the future us.

They were asking themselves what I would do at a time or moment of a racial slur. Will I know what is being said and how to handle it. Have I ever seen a naked woman, any part of her body being exposed on a phone or physically in front of me. They also got to the simplest thing; like will I be able to recognize a scent that is not pleasant.

I would say this, they did not ponder these thoughts in the past because the idea of college for me did not come about until my junior year of high school. So, it never occurred to them to ask the simplest questions. This was to only believe that they did enough as would any other parent for that matter.

Now, I have been beckoned to join in on the conversations. Once I got outside with them, my father started the questions and I calmly listened to him as his voice conjures your attention. I would think that now I had all the right answers; but how many of you know that even the right answers are wrong?

When ask, have you ever seen a woman without her clothing, fully naked. When your answer is no, I think he would have wanted me to say yes. This was only to say that now I have been exposed, then maybe it would be easy to explain it to me.

"Expectations"

When he got the answer, he now must find a way in his heart and mind to explain to me how it is not right to embark upon such shame. Unless it is in a time of fulfillment of one's desires and both parties agree. We would want the road traveled in this case, to better wrap our minds around this idea opposed to the less traveled option.

They would have possibly preferred that I had already experienced such a thing, but I'm sorry to be disappointed. While still in this uncomfortable position, feeling overwhelmed with their questions, I knew in my mind they were necessary.

There were other questions, especially with the racism thoughts that may or may not come to me. They just gave me bits of this to help me easily identify when the non-welcoming verbiage came my way, what it would sound like. How I should respond, had they come in such a manner.

They also elaborated that these are conversations that many of our culture must have today to keep ourselves safe. To make sure that we are not in vulnerable situations, I mean just wide open and subjective to such activity. In other words, stay focused, pay attention to your company, and know who is among you.

Here is where my mother would jump in and give me a scenario. She said, "What if we were not out here on the porch with you. There was a female walking right in front of you in the parking lot and she was naked, what would you do?"

It took me a moment to get my thoughts around the question, but they were very proud of my response. I said, "I would come and get you and dad." She came back with, "What would you then say for us to respond to?" I said, "Mom there is a young lady outside naked."

My mother cried and my dad just gave a gentle smile and nodded his head. It was in those moments and responses that he and my mother realized that I was going to be alright. That they could put their hearts at ease because I am good, and God will carry me the rest of the way.

Monumental moments with great expectations always bring great joy and solace. These are the tilling of the soil inserts to my growth and where I am headed. The shattering of stigmas and pressing toward greater instances will be a growing moment for me. They are so defining what is destined for

Exceptional

my journey and how I will capitalize on the trials and tribulations that will shape me into who I am in the future.

I have found that the less I believe in disability and seek out greatness, the more I have nothing to lose but everything to gain. Expecting what some say is "exceptional" and others say extraordinary!

This is not to say that my parents will not continue to have some doubts, it is only to say even in the doubts they still push me to better. They want to see what was already shown to them, the very thing that is beautiful and pure is just and absolute!

The champion inside of them that never gave in or quit, it is in my sister and me. It is passed on from them to us and then onto our children and so on!

It is all generational and because they sought for the generational curses to stop with them, we get to swim in the benefits of it all. We get to tell our children, if we have any at all, that we see different and we experience new and great.

The story is being rewritten with all the richness and tears and pain life has to offer. The story that is being told now has more expectations. They are the kind of expectations that will live on to build legacies and take over territory that was not taken by our previous ancestors.

This was not because they did not want these things for themselves, it was because they did only what they were exposed to and knew. The limits were not due to knowledge but more so to exposure, because without that, how do you know?

In this writing, I can only take you as far my age at this time will allow. I am in my teen years ready to set ablaze the path that has been paved for me. To seek out what is predestined for a lad such as myself. I too have my anxieties of what this next chapter is going to look like, but even in that, I am ready.

My expectations alone brought me to this point of transition, and I am walking on to see the manifestation of such a thing. Before I expound on anything else and move on to the next big thing, please elaborate on your expectations for yourself and those around you as they contribute.

Expectations Journal

What are your expectations from here?

What exactly may have you stuck and feeling like quitting?

Does someone else's opinion of you now or your past has damaged your possibilities?

How long will you allow such thoughts to continue to construct your future?

Exceptional

Is there anyone or anything that inspires you? Who, what, and why?
___
___
___
___
___

CHAPTER 7
"RESHAPING"

Timeless moments are unpredictable. They are stumbled upon with much anticipation, like where and how the wind comes and goes while stretching the imagination. Pouring water into a glass that has no base, while wanting to escape and hoping time spent was not a waste.

The formation of my thoughts comes jumbled but with the love that helps me to unfold, keeps me humbled. We stand in a space that seems to be empty, yet as time evolves, I say Father, be with me.

Searching for another part of me, to envision a future with love, companionship with strong desire. I too am no different than to take time and navigate with caution, with hopes to inspire and admire.

I come to paint the canvas of my life, to prepare the meal that I want to feast upon. Delivering to the world a savory, mouthwatering phenomenon. Only time will tell where anyone goes and why? The participating villagers dare only to say fly eagle fly!

Taking this journey and calling it beautiful, has only given me superpowers. The way around this is to imagine it can be done within hours. As I am challenged to see it no other way, life tells me otherwise.

My future has this physical aspect call eyes and I see it reaching many others to change their perspectives. It is this innate ability to know you only get what you can think or believe that tells me so. It allows me to see the past where I am currently and achieve great things.

Stretch yourself for the unthinkable, unimaginable, and uncompromising. I dare you to dream, and when you do, if you are not scared; watch the distance on the road with less resistance.

Take the leap, it might be steep, but forward movement is why our heart still beats. Join yourself as you journey, this may sound like it is only for me, but you too are a part of this. I promise you; your future self does not want you to miss this.

Filling

When this is all said and done, you would not want to look back with regrets. None that will have you wanting to give up on life and not see anything good that was of a promising deed. The way I see it, we could allow others to come in and take away and not give, but this is totally up to us.

I know, you might say, well I cannot really think for myself, well if you just had that thought then you can think for yourself. I know I crack my own self up at times and wonder am I truly trapped or plagued by what the world may say of me. These are thoughts even the average person would think upon.

In the later years of my life, I am not sure of what they would look like. I am not even sure if I would get to enjoy them. While I think about it, I want nothing more than to be at my own future parties and gatherings with family and friends. So, "yes," I have no other choice but to push through the noise.

We cannot make everyone happy with who we are and what we become, but we can surely be glad that we have even made it. I have my parents to thank for much of this kind of thinking, along with my sister, my nephew, and my brother in love Enock. I did not talk much about my nephew, only because I don't believe that I am going to be the same by the time he is a teen.

I look forward to the growth of my time here on earth, with everything that it has to offer, same or indifferent. I would like to suggest one thing to you all; being different is not a bad thing. If you really look at this word, "different," we all fall under this definition.

I mean, every one of us on the planet falls under this word. Seriously, if God created us all to be the same, well I would not want to even be on the planet with a whole bunch of me running around. This would truly be the blind leading the blind.

We must simply embrace our differences, be a positive asset to society, and grow in that very thing. There is truly not enough lifting, there is more tearing down than anything. This is ranging from our homes and family to politics and economical ideologies.

If we only understood more of how we are all needed to grow, stand, become, and change the world; then we will have seen and experienced true love. The very word that matters the most and only one that matters is "love!"

My mother said, this word is composed of one syllable, and it has four letters, and it is the hardest thing for people to display. Not all have issues with this word, only the ones that say it without any weight to it.

We have become so complacent with this word that it just comes off our lips with ease and has no truth to it anymore. We have killed, lied, and stolen because of this one word. To me it is the most powerful word out of all of Webster's dictionary, yet the one least valued.

If you say this word, it requires action as it is a verb, it is the act of caring and giving to someone else according to the dictionary. I mean how can you do this or say this when first you may not feel the same way about yourself.

That is like telling someone to ask you, I have one hundred dollars to give you, but you do not have it. So how then can you say or do this to another and not have it? Well, let me enlighten you with that answer.

With all the hurt and damage in the mind and hearts of the people, they are truly empty vessels walking around giving this word out for free. It has no value anymore, and we have done this by allowing hurt and unforgiveness to come into our being. It is because of that you should know that love is greater and the only thing that matters.

As this is the greatest gift that God has given to us freely by and because of the death of his only Son. It is because of Him that I get to write this to you and allow you a way towards greater and better. So just know it is not over for you and your different self, it is only just beginning.

There is this saying in Italian that I learned while over in Italy that meant so much to me. It has also been used within the movie, *Eat Pray Love*. The saying is not the word love, but it tells us how to do this thing call, relax and enjoy life. It is ever so potent within itself and universal.

The words are, *"Dolce farniente."* It simply means sweetness of doing nothing, pleasantness.[10] Only if we could sit back and see the benefits come in after our laboring, then and only then will we exude love for ourselves and others.

I cannot express enough how we really need to reevaluate this word and the proven power of it. Once we have done that, we can go out and possess the land. I do not mean the land as the one we walk upon, but the souls of the people and having them to capture the full essence of life.

This will allow for greater expansion and resolve to change the thoughts and minds of ourselves first and others that are connected to us. I long for this beautiful revelation and how it will one day be the blanketing effect of changed minds and renewed lives.

"Reshaping"

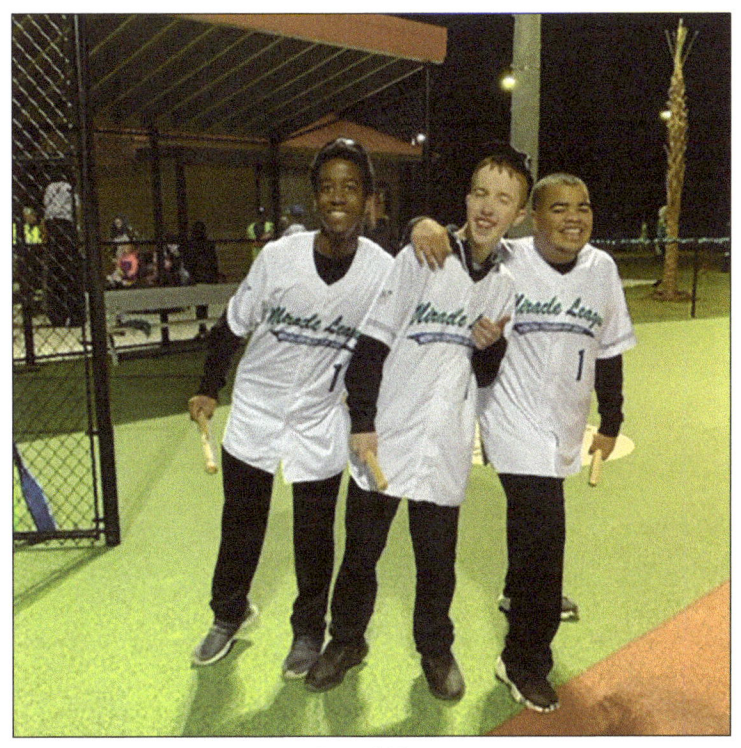

C2 and Trey

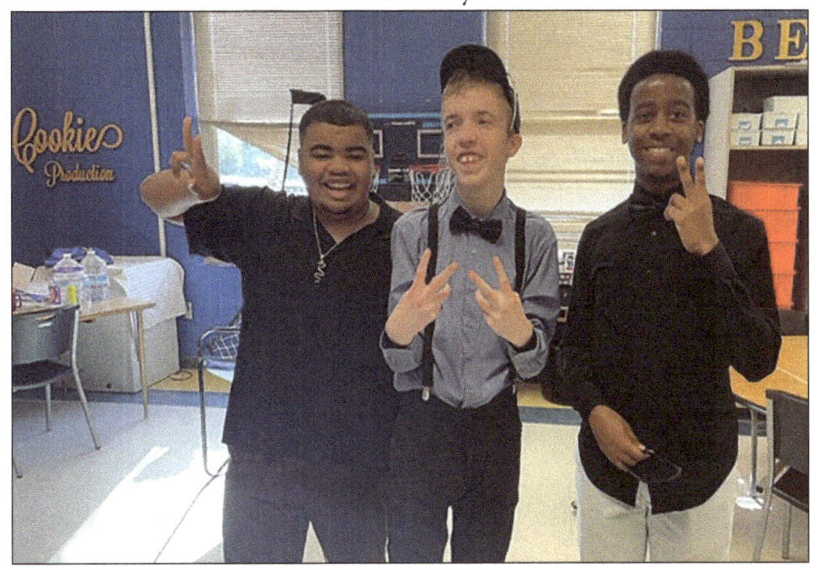

Trey and Carl (my friends for life)

Exceptional

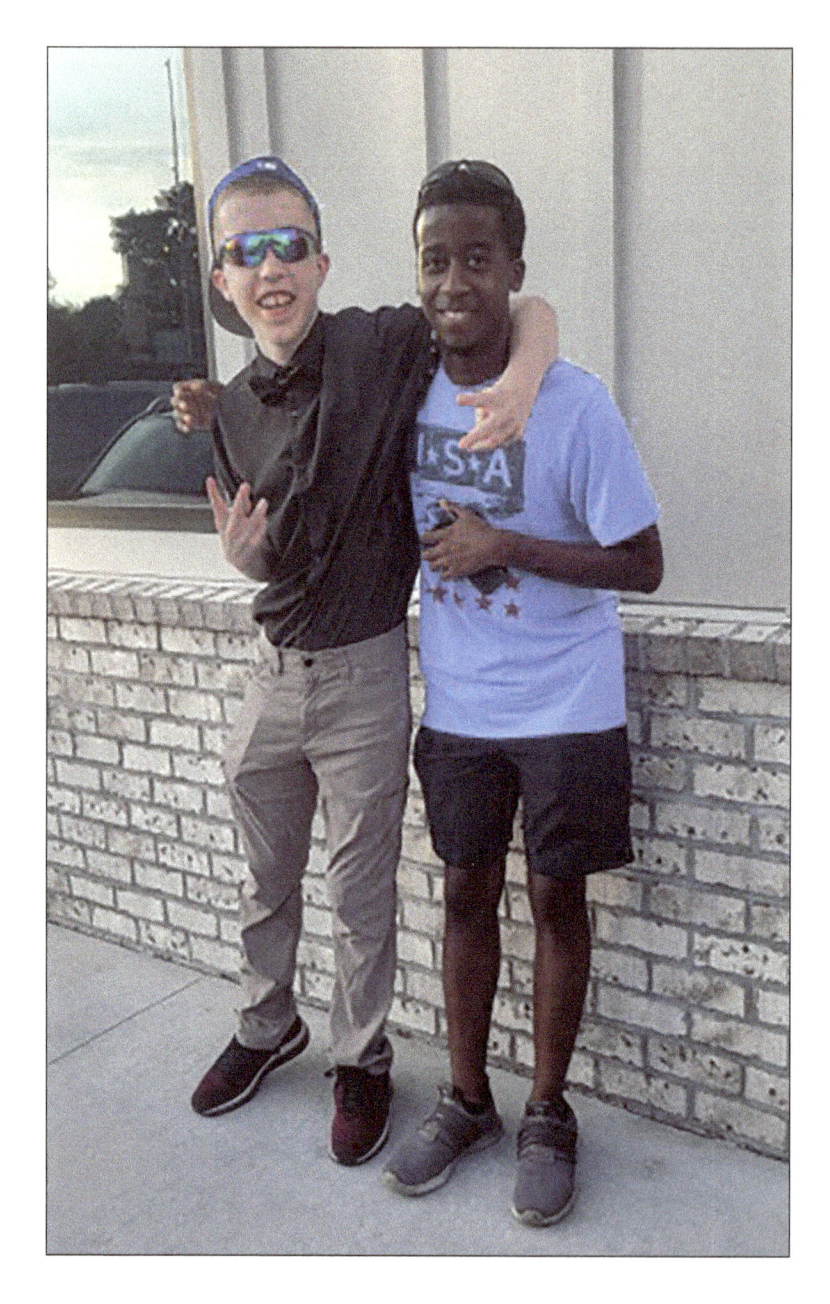

Carl Sole A.K.A. C2

CONCLUSION

Words have no power unless we believe in what is being said. Also, having the mindset to take the words out of context makes belief more difficult. People are going to say what they want to say and however they desire to do so. It is totally up to us how we perceive what is being said and how they deliver it.

The word Autism or ASD is truly just a word that has a definition and meaning. It does not mean that it must be our defining truth. The truth is, we are fearfully and wonderfully made! We have been so ostracized by the world and defined by terms that we have simply lost our identity.

We are no longer being defined by what we believe ourselves to be, we allow someone else to define us. This will not help us to defy the odds, it will only prevent us from meeting our real self. The true us that we have been predestined to become and effect change.

I am not saying that the diagnosis is not fact, it is, I am asking you what is the truth? How will you allow what has been diagnosed to define you? Will you simply roll over in this and surrender? Will the symptoms be the definition for a permanent outcome or a pressing outbreak?

How long does the frustration in your world and mind carry on before you intervene and say, "enough is enough!" We are truly much more powerful within ourselves than we can ever imagine. The shame will not be the thing that is placed on us, it will be the regrets of, "what if, I should have and could have."

Why do this to yourself when your inner spirit is fighting for more common ground and peace? Imagine that we are at an intersection and those that are at this point of change, are all different. There is nothing

Exceptional

wrong with us all being there at the same time, we all will simply go in different directions.

This gives way to understanding, even though we may arrive at the same thing, we are still different and all going in different directions. We are still exceptional beings, striving for giant outcomes to cease the moments that are presented to us.

Alright, this is the most profound of this entire writing. I had the opportunity to see the beauty of checking in, arriving, and getting settled into college life. I had gained some confidence in the last few days to separate from my parents and family. There came the time to sever the line of birth from my mother.

We pulled up to Clemson University on August 20, 2023, only to find the most amazing, and beautiful display of people and their excellence! I mean my mother and my father could not be more pleased and moved by their welcome for us. This I would believe gave my parents ease to leave me behind.

They both exited the vehicle and the team that they had now communicated with via email would now really display their excellence in full capacity. It was invigorating and pulsating all in the same breath. They could not be more pleased or expected anything less from the best program in all the United States.

I on the other hand was ready for what was next in this thrill and with some sadness that my mother saw in my eyes gave her some sadness as well. We both knew these days were coming, but now they are here! We all needed these moments and days to come, but we had the happy and sad feelings in it all.

The way someone can feel happy for the mountain top experience and still have this valley feeling of sadness and some depression. The pain and discomfort will persist within my mother as she would now have to go home and leave me. She would soon feel the drought of expression, kisses, sounds and other emotions of me not being around. There is this transitional period here at Clemson during which we cannot communicate with our parents, and it was very hard. It was hard for my mother not to hear my voice, feel my kiss, or my arms around her.

Conclusion

She stated that she felt like she could not breathe and almost had an anxiety attack from all the emotional bomb rushing. It was like someone had ripped off a large bandage from her back and left a huge wound. She said there was a moment when she awoke the next morning, that she did not hear me say good morning and that was so painful for her.

She longed so for these days and wanted to come and get me so she could then keep the luxury of me being near her and with her. I can understand all of this. How now I needed them and to depend on their mind, heart, spirit, and soul to grow and care for me, but now I get to fly.

I remember her saying, "can I sleep with him in his dorm room over this last night?" She asked my instructor this question and she laughed, but my mother was so for real. I know this would be some strange, beautiful phenomenon but in the end, it is all worth it. Go Tigers!

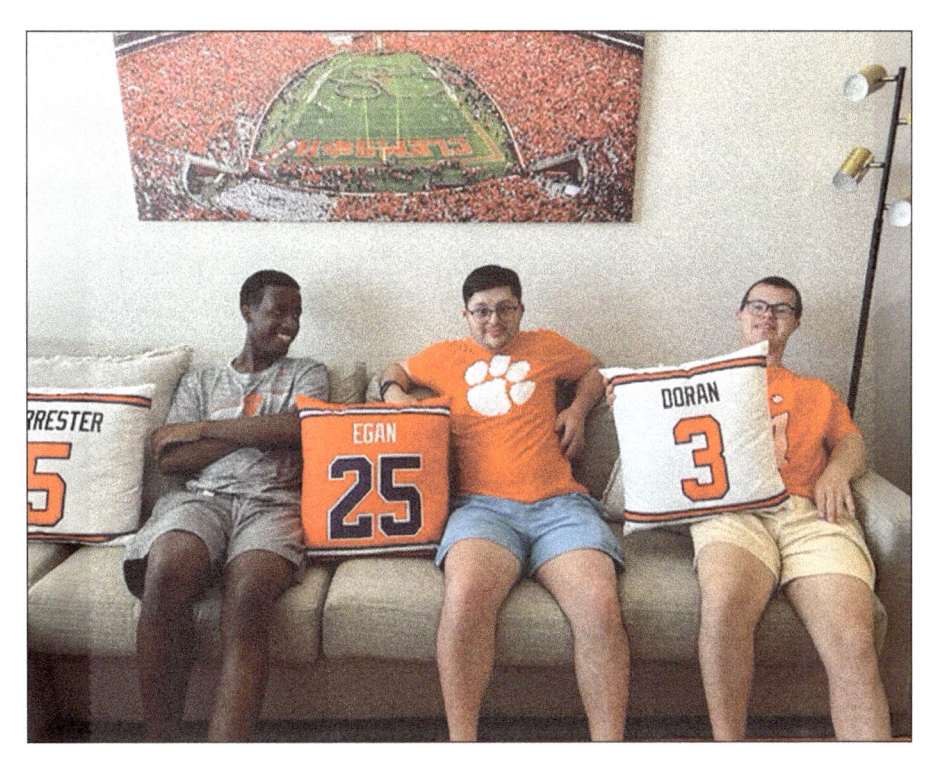

Zylin Forrester at Clemson University
"Go Tigers!"

"Journey well my gentle souls and see what the end will be."

Exceptional

The pages of this book have been breathtaking to say the least, but all so powerful. I know that I have just started my life living beyond the walls and definition of my parents. I now get to see past the mountain with hopes of having that top experience while the valley is present as well.

I will be excellent; I will have that one wife and the beauty of children one day. The career path that some may not have seen for me, but I knew of it all along. The visions were there, now I am pressing toward the provisions of it all.

Thank you all for being a part of Exceptional and seeing extraordinary! I applaud and praise my future, for it will be great and you can join in for yours as well!

Beautiful beginnings with expected endings!
"Beaux debuts avec des fins attendues!"

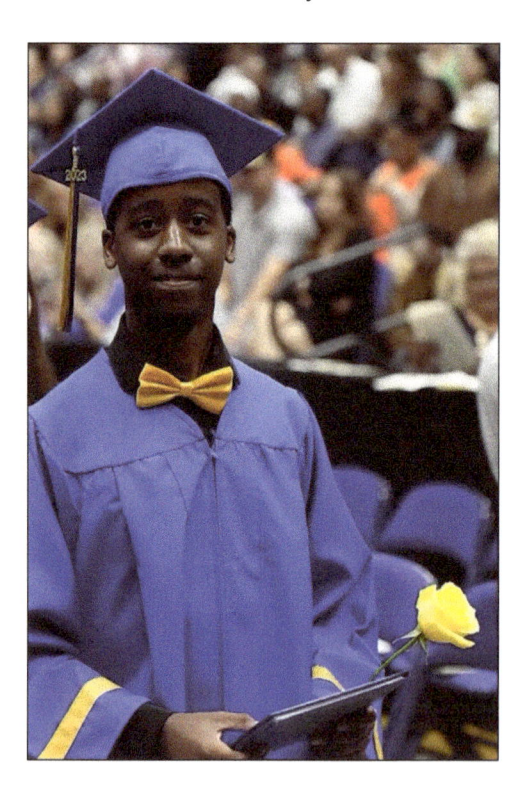

Conclusion

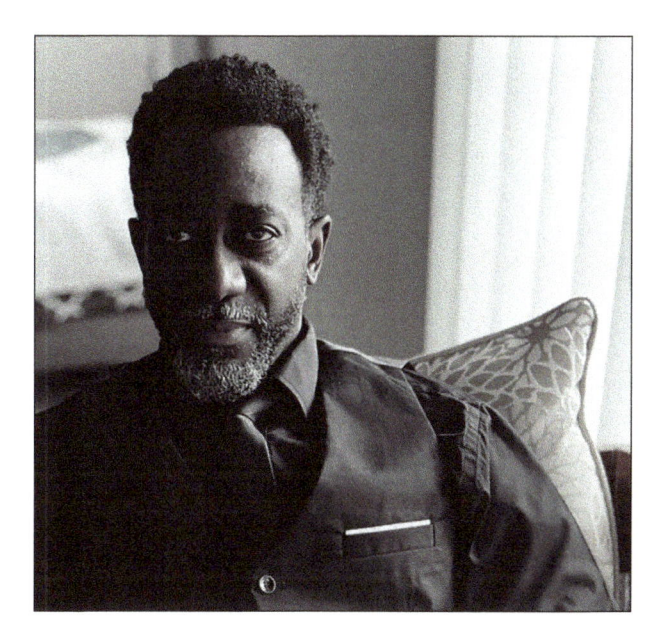

My Dad

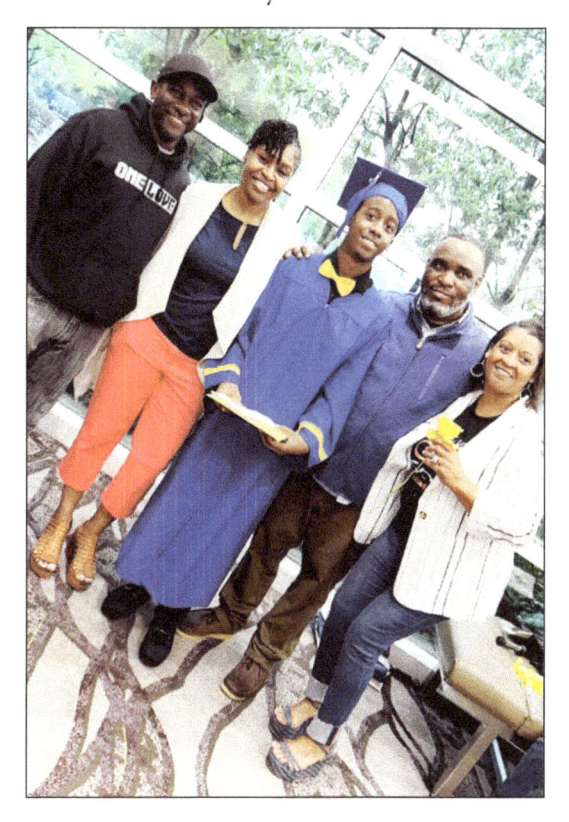

Exceptional

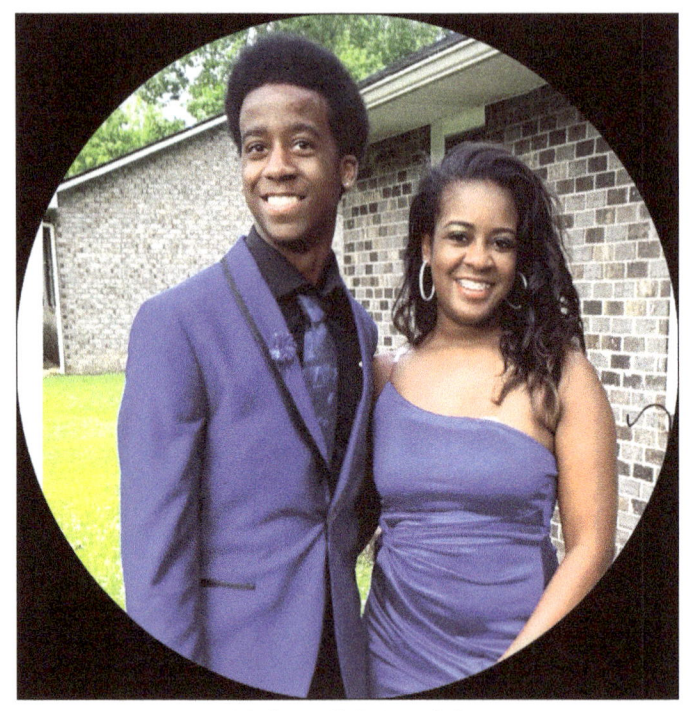

My beautiful sister & I

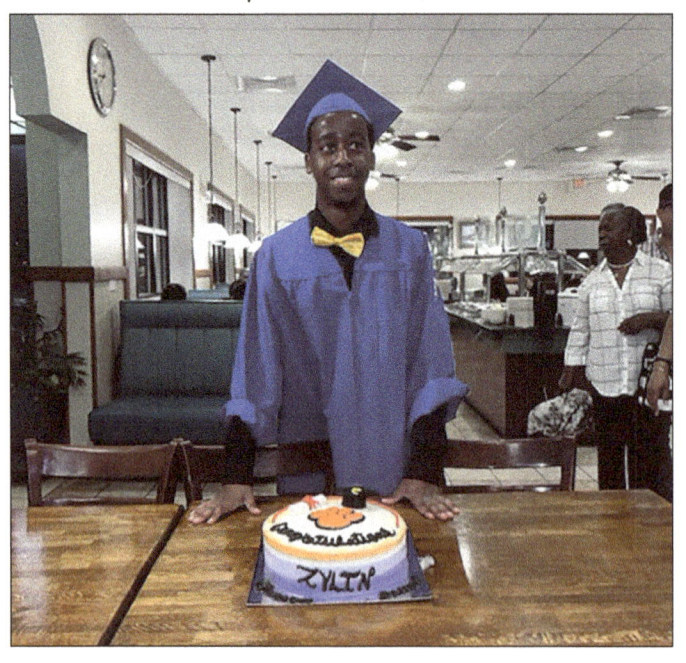

Conclusion

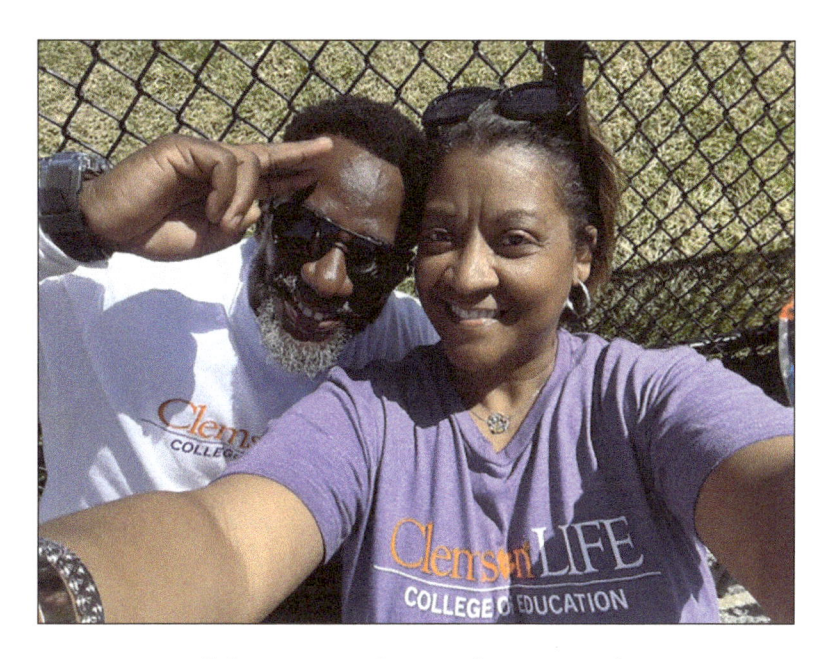

"Clemson For Life Parents" Mom & Dad

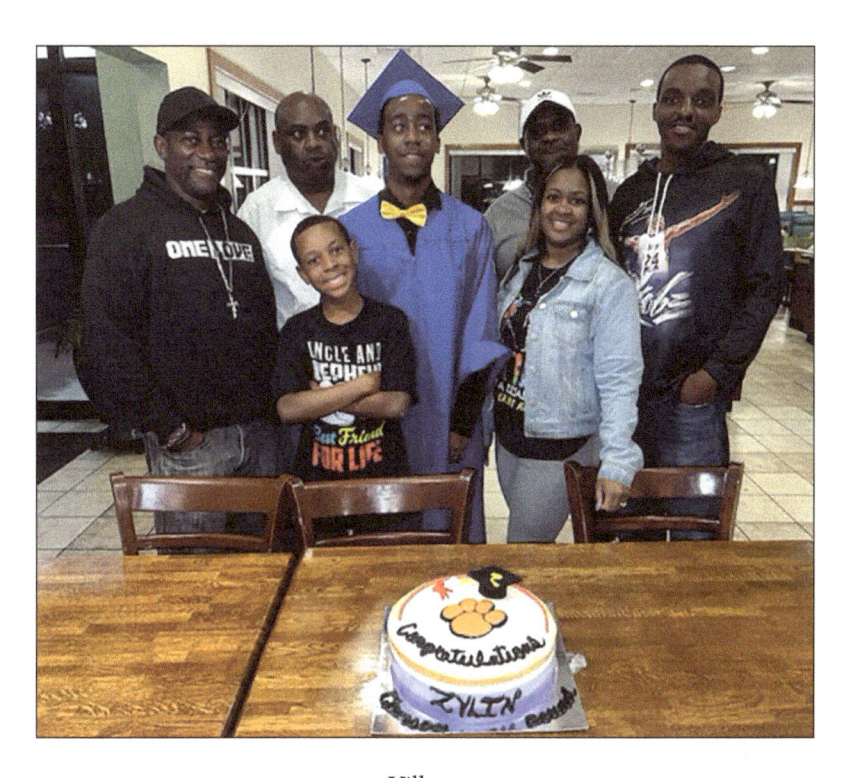

Village

ABOUT THE AUTHOR

ANNETTE FORRESTER is the voice behind this book and the mother to the Co-Author of this book. She is a resident of Charleston, South Carolina, by way of Estill South Carolina. Annette is the wife of 20 years to Alfonso Forrester. She is also a veteran with 12 years of service for the United States Army. Annette has also completed her Certification with the University of Purdue Global in Health and Human Services. She did not stop there, she has also completed a Certification in Massage Therapy, with Miller Motte Technical College in North Charleston, South Carolina. Annette graduated from Miller Motte with honors of Summa Cum Laude. Annette has since gone on to pursue her dreams of becoming an Author, giving way to her first book "Hidden" The Anatomy of Healing, being published in May of 2022. Annette is now partnering with her son to shine light on "Autism," and its journey within our communities. Since, the writing of "Hidden," she was featured in her local magazine "Charleston Women," within their May/June edition. Now, with the journey of writing and becoming a best seller author, she is excited for what the future holds and endeavors for business.

ABOUT THE CO-AUTHOR

ZYLIN FORRESTER is the son of Alfonso and Annette Forrester, of Estill, South Carolina. He was born in Vicenza, Italy by way of the Armed Forces. He was diagnosed with autism spectrum disorder when he was four years of age in Hawaii. Zylin has also served his community by volunteering at CLM (Changed Life Ministries) in Moncks Corner South Carolina. Zylin is a High School graduate of Berkeley High School of Moncks Corner, South Carolina class of 2023. Zylin has been accepted within the L.I.F.E program at Clemson University for the fall of 2023. Zylin's dream was to attend Clemson and their L.I.F.E (Learning Is for Everyone) program to gain access to a better way of life while living with Autism. This dream has since come true. Once He completes this program, he then looks to obtain a degree in Dental Hygiene and possibly Music Therapy. Zylin will continue to pursue whatever is next for him and his family, to ensure that he is a great asset to society.

ABOUT THE AUTHORS

Annette was born and raised in Estill, South Carolina to the late John Henry Busby and Jaenell Busby. Annette is the wife to Alfonso Forrester and mother to the co-author Zylin Forrester. Annette is a veteran of the United States Army after serving 12 years of service. Annette took it upon herself to continue her education to become a certified Massage Therapist in 2013 through Miller Motte Technical College of North Charleston, South Carolina. She also went on to pursue her career path with a certification in Health and Human Services, graduating from Purdue Global University. She looks forward to what is next for her family and writing career. She is also the author of "Hidden" The Anatomy of Healing, which was released in May of 2022.

Zylin was born in Vicenza, Italy on August 5, 2005, to Alfonso and Annette Forrester. While his mother served within the Armed Forces, he was new to the land and world of Italy. Zylin was born with some major birth delays. He started out with seizures during his 6-month-old to 7 years of age time frame. Zylin endured much while in such young years of his life. Once Zylin turned 4 years old, he was diagnosed with Autism. This was the start of new roads to journey for Zylin and his family. Zylin went on to attend school in several different states and has since graduated from Berkeley High School of Moncks Corner, South Carolina. He has gained some great ground with new friends and overcame many obstacles. Since Zylin's graduation from High School, he has been accepted in the LIFE (Learning is For Everyone) program at Clemson University, of Clemson, South Carolina. Zylin will be attending their fall semester starting in August of 2023. Zylin looks

Exceptional

forward to you capturing the beauty of this book and all that it will display for those alike. *"Bellissimo!"*

ACKNOWLEDGMENTS

I want to take this time to acknowledge my mother for her great gifts. First of her being a mother to me and my sibling. I love her for all that she does and say to keep me in the right standing with God and all those that are connected to me. She is the queen to my father and my beautiful star that will always shine brightly in my heart.

Also, to thank my loving father! He is a king to my mother and the stability to my standing with much vigor and vitality. He has grown and displayed such a firm belief in God after his transformation in life. With his strength and my mother's elegance, I am thankful that I do not have to search for love, because it woke up with me, fed me, taught me, and now it has propelled me too greater! Thanks Dad, my rock and hero!

To my sister, my beautiful, strong, and of great courage of a woman; you exemplify the definition of fortitude! You have not always been so fond of me but grew into loving me even though you were no longer the only child. I know I came along and threw your entire life in a frenzy. Look at it this way sis, now we get to experience some of the greatest parents ever!!! We can share in the love that they have and once we both reach greatness in life, we can then take care of them. I Love you! *"Bella!"*

To my nephew! Yes, saving the best for last! I truly cannot say enough about you and how you grow more and more. This is to say, how your ways have helped me to see how I should act as a young man. You were not always nice to me, but I did get you back with my pushing and shoving on you. While you were sometimes unwelcoming, I still love you and always will. I can't wait until you depend on me and not so much, I depend on you. I Love you nephew!

Exceptional

To my god parents and siblings! Here is where I get to enjoy the luxury of having two sets of parents. I mean what more can anyone ask for than to have so much love being poured into you. I really am thankful and grateful that my parents accepted you to see me as more than a memory. You took it upon yourselves to love me as your own and I will always respect and cherish the moments shared and times to come. *"One love!"*

Enock! Our new addition to the family. You came along with your smoothness and charismatic demeanor, to help with my growth as a man. To add to what my father may lack to give. All people add to our lives rather we want to believe it or not, but they really do. Some in times take away and do it without any regard for what they may have caused. With you, there is a great addition and now we can cut it up as you allow me space to see what a brother should look like and be. I will always pray for your healing and growth. *Je t'aime!*

To all my church family past and present! What can I say when God has orchestrated such a divine move to see growth and maturity. I truly respect and honor the people of God and all that he has allowed for me during my time with all, currently the Place of Prayer Tabernacle. With the disciples that God is grooming and growing under such an awesome and powerful Bishop and Pastor. I thank you all for your love, donations, encouraging words to help me along the way. I especially, want to thank Bishop Torrest Richardson and Pastor Darlene Richardson, for helping me navigate through my thoughts and dreams. You are both great for this season, and I truly pray that God continues to shine his light upon you all with overflow and abundance. Love you all POP church!

The best friends of mine! To the coolest dudes on the east coast and how they get me, and I get them. Listen, without you guys and the conversations we have had, I would have to say that I would not have anyone in my phone contacts. I truly respect our friendship and how we can relate to each other and find cool things to talk about while hanging out together. We might be leaving each other behind and going in our own ways, but we will not lose conversations! Big ups to Trey and Carl.

Acknowledgments

I also thank your parents for trusting us as a family to hang out and converse. Thank you all! My brothers from another mother!

A special thanks to Chelsea Swanier for her gift and skills of photography. Blessings and overflow.

REFERENCES

1. "Autism spectrum disorder (ASD)," Autism Speaks, https://www.autismspeaks.org/what-autism.

2. Center for Disease Control, n.d., https://www.cdc.com.

3. "DSM-5 and autism: Frequently asked questions," Autism Speaks, https://www.autismspeaks.org/dsm-5-and-autism-frequently-asked-questions.

4. Dr. Ananya Mandal and April Cashin-Garbutt, MA (ed.), "Autism History," *News Medical*, last updated July 7, 2023, https://www.news-medical.net/health/Autism-History.aspx.

5. "The History Of Autism: Science, Research, And Progress," ABA Centers of America, March 25, 2022, https://www.abacenters.com/history-of-autism/.

6. Isobel (Izzy) Mulkern, "Autism: Symbols to Remember," Twinkl, https://www.twinkl.com/blog/autism-symbols-to-remember.

7. John Harris, "The mother of neurodiversity: how Judy Singer changed the world," *The Guardian*, July 5, 2023, https://www.theguardian.com/world/2023/jul/05/the-mother-of-neurodiversity-how-judy-singer-changed-the-world.

8. *Wonder*, directed by Stephen Chbosky (2017, Santa Monica, CA: Lions Gate Entertainment Corporation, 2018).

Exceptional

9. "expectation," *Merriam-Webster.com Dictionary*, https://www.merriam-webster.com/dictionary/expectation.

11. *Eat Pray Love,* directed by Ryan Murphy (2010, Culver City, CA and Beverly Hills, CA: Columbia Pictures and Plan B. Entertainment, 2010).